CREATIVITY AND COGNITIVE STYLES IN CHILDREN

A. KUSUMA

M.Sc., M.Ed., M.Phil., P.G. Dip. in Statistics, Ph.D.

Department of Human Development and Family Studies,
Sri Padmavathi Mahila Visvavidyalayam,
Tirupati (A.P.)

DISCOVERY PUBLISHING HOUSE

NEW DELHI—110 002

Reprinted - 2018
First Published - 1997

ISBN: 978-81-7141-333-1

Creativity and Cognitive Styles in Children

Published by:
DISCOVERY PUBLISHING HOUSE PVT. LTD.
4383/4B, Ansari Road, Darya Ganj
New Delhi-110 002 (India)
Phone: +91-11-23279245, 43596064-65
Fax: +91-11-23253475
E-mail: discoverypublishinghouse@gmail.com
sales@discoverypublishinggroup.com
web: www.discoverypublishinggroup.com

Printed at:
Infinity Imaging Systems
Delhi

ACKNOWLEDGEMENTS

With great respect and due reverence, I express my deep sense of gratitude and indebtedness to my guide Dr. S.R. Venkatramaiah, Professor of Clinical Psychology, Department of Home Science, Sri Venkateswara University, Tirupati, for the guidance and encouragement he has given me throughout this investigation. I deem it a great and rare privilege for having got the opportunity of working under him.

I am most indebted to Prof. Ms. P.R. Reddy, Vice-chancellor, Sri Padmavathi Mahila Viswavidyalayam, Tirupati, for her encouragement, advise and valuable suggestions given through out the study.

I am thankful to Ms. K. Chandralekha, Head, Department of Home Science, S.V. University, Tirupati for administrative support.

I express my sincere thanks to Dr. V. Kodanda Rami Reddy, Reader, Department of Econometrics, S.V. University, Tirupati, for computerising the data.

I profoundly thank Mrs. V. Vijayalakshmi, Lecturer, Department of Home Science, S.V. University, Tirupati, for her valuable assistance in expediting the statistical part of the thesis work.

My thanks are also due to the teaching and non-teaching staff members of the department of Home Science, S.V. University, Tirupati, for their assistance from time to time to complete this research work.

I am highly indebted to my parents and husband, Dr. G. Lokanadha Reddy, Lecturer, Department of Education, Alagappa University, Karaikudi, who were a constant source of encouragement and moral support in my career.

I wish to thank the Head Masters/Mistresses, Teachers and Students of selected schools for extending their co-operation while collecting the data.

My thanks are due to Mr. M. Nagaraju, for typing this thesis very neatly and quickly.

I also thank the friends and well-wishers for their help in successful completion of the thesis.

A. Kusuma

FOREWORD

Progress in varied dimensions like economic growth, technological development and psychological well-being of a nation rests basically upon the creative talents and appropriate cognitive styles of individuals.

When we look critically the present day educational practice, one of the laccunae is a lack of importance given to creativity. So it is necessary to generate research data on creativity and performance where excellence is given highest premium. The performance and attainment of a child in the present educational system depends very much upon perceptual growth and efficient cognitive styles. To see the impact of cognitive styles on intellectual and academic achievements basically the research is needed on cognitive styles.

There are a few books relating to creativity and cognitive styles in children. Further, books focusing how certain demographic psychological and environmental factors contributes to the expression of creativity and cognitive styles employed in dealing with the external world are very meagre. In this context, the book in your hands entitled "Creativity and Cognitive Styles in Children" is written by Dr. A. Kusuma, Lecturer, Dept. of Human Development and Family Studies, Sri Padmavathi Mahila Visvavidyalayam, Tirupati, Andhra Pradesh. This book is a significant attempt in highlighting the verbal and non-verbal components of creativity and field dependence/independence, reflection/impulsivity cognitive styles in tribal and non-tribal children.

The present book is a highly useful source and helpful research compendium for the teachers, teacher educators, programme planners, administrators, researchers and students working in the field of Home Science, Education, Psychology and allied disciplines.

Prof. A. Satyavathi
Principal
University College
Sri Padmavathi Mahila Visvavidyalayam,
Tirupati, Andhra Pradesh.

CONTENTS

CONTENTS

1

INTRODUCTION

> **"Our children are the pillars of the nation and they must be cared for and protected at all costs, under suitable environment."**
>
> **—Jawaharlal Nehru**

The children of the world are innocent, vulnerable and dependent. They are also curious, active and full of hope. Their time should be full of joy and peace, a period of playing, learning and growing. Their future should be shaped in harmony and cooperation. Their lives should mature as they broaden their perspectives and gain new experiences (UNICEF, 1991).

According to UNICEF (1991) in India, nearly 324.5 million children are under 16 years of age who are the future citizens of the nation.

The majority of children in India are underprivileged. They live under low social, economic and environmental conditions which hamper their growth and development. Many families live at the subsistence level and are plagued with illiteracy and unemployment. As put forth by UNICEF (1983) the problem relating to child care and development are therefore complex.

In post-independent India, the political ideal of democratic socialism is committed to the protection and all-round development

of the people belonging to weaker sections of society. The scheduled castes and scheduled tribes fall under this category of weaker sections. Anthropologists have found difficult to develop a set of precise indices to distinguish tribals from non-tribals. But, broadly speaking, the term refers to territorial communities, the bulk of whom live in the isolation of hills and forests. They are integrated in terms of certain themes rooted in the past. Their distinct cultural focus gives them a separate identity.

An ethnic group may be defined as group of individuals with a shared sense of peoplehood (Gordon, 1964) based on presumed shared socio-cultural experiences and for similar physical characteristics. Such groups may be viewed by their members and/or outsiders as religious, racial, national, linguistic and/or geographical. Thus, what ethnic group members have in common is their ethnicity or sense of peoplehood, which represents a part of their collective experience.

SOME RELEVANT CONCEPTS AND ISSUES

Ethnicity and Cognitive Development

Socialization goals stemming from adaptive strategies of ethnic group families influence children's cognitive development. The socialization process is complex and it is difficult to ascribe development outcomes to specific factors. The research evidence for these and similar questions is diffuse, sparse, uneven across ethnic groups and lacking for some (McShane, 1988), yet some insights can be gleaned from the general literature on ethnic group children and families. Within-group differences are an important source of variance when studying developmental outcomes on child behavioural measures. Investigators have examined the variables of social class (Carter, 1983; DeVos, 1973; Hakuta, 1987 and Shon and Ja, 1983), identification with ethnic culture (Buriel, 1984 and McShane, 1983), generation status (Buriel, Calzada and Vasques, 1982), geographic origin (Shon and Ja, 1983), father absence (Powell, et al., 1983 and scott-Jones, 1987), gender (Hare and Castenell, 1985), home environment (Slaughter and Epps, 1987) and geographical habitats (McShane and Berry, 1986) as examples of important determinants of intragroup heterogeneity.

Theories abound explaining the determinants, course, and trends of cognitive development. Currently, the concepts of Vygotsky (1978) are receiving increased attention as a framework for investigating the importance of culture to cognitive development. Vygotsky viewed children as active participants who attempted to master and competently function in the world around them. One of the ways they mastered their world was through the use of auxiliary stimuli. Auxiliary stimuli are introduced as a means of active adaptation and include the tools of the culture into which the child is born, the language of those who relate to the child, and other means produced by the child. Thus, Vygotsky concluded that in order to study development in children, one must begin with an understanding of two principally different entities, the biological and the cultural.

The ideas of Vygotsky (1978) have been expanded and serve as a source of fresh insights in the area of developmental psychology (e.g., Irvine and Berry, 1986). Bronfenbrenner (1989) summarized the essence of this trend as proposing that the attributes of the person most likely to shape the beginning of the course of one's cognitive development are those that induce or inhibit dynamic dispositions toward the immediate environment, referred to as developmentally instigative characteristics.

Researchers have consistently found that ethnic group families are concerned with biculturalism or preparing children to function in both the ethnic and non-ethnic communities (Harrison, et al., 1984 and Peters, 1988). Theoretical and empirical evidence (Ramirez, 1983) indicates that biculturalism often involves more than using two cultural modalities in a simple additive manner (Gutierrez, et al., 1988). The process of integrating two cultural systems involves grater cognitive and social flexibility that eventuates in a unique synthesis of both ethnic and non-ethnic cultures as well as separateness of both cultures. Achieving the new synthesis is a complex process fraught with many obstacles and conflicts.

Biculturalism can be expressed in values, identity and customs. Nevertheless, bilingualism is perhaps the most investigated indicator (Hakuta and Garcia, 1989). Balanced bilingual children show more cognitive flexibility than monolingual children (McShane and Berry, 1986; McShane and Cook, 1985; Osborne, 1985; Ramirez and Castaneda, 1974 and Seifert and Hoffnung, 1985), that is, the ability to detect multiple meanings of words and alternative orientations of objects. Studies also indicate that bilingualism fosters metalinguistic awareness, the cognitive ability to attend to language as an object of thought rather than just for the content or idea (Diaz, 1983).

Discontinuity has been defined as an abrupt transition from one mode of being and behaving to another accompanied by noticeable differences in social role assignments and expectations (Marcias, 1987). The problems generated by discontinuity between the home environments of ethnic group children and the school environment are of concern. Discontinuity has the possibility of negative consequences on cognitive functioning because it affects academic achievement and social adjustment (Osborne, 1985 and Spindler and Spindler, 1987). Ethnic group children are more likely to be exposed to discontinuities between their family ecologies and school environment than non-ethnic group children. Continuity between learning environments of home and school is an important element in the performance of children on problem - solving tasks (Delgado - Gaitan, 1987; Lasoa and Sigel, 1982 and Marcias, 1987). Research studies have found that ethnic group children show improvements in their achievement levels memory, and problem-solving abilities when the context of the learning environment is consistent with their background (Boykin, 1979; Hare, 1985; Holliday, 1985 and spindler and Spindler, 1987). This phenomenon is highlighted in the teaching strategies, parents use in interactions with their children. The teaching/learning strategies used in the home influences how children perform on problem-solving situations in school (Laosa, 1980; Laosa and Deavila, 1979 and Steward and Steward, 1973).

Theoretical Background Of Cognitive Development

Werner (1947) believes in common developmental principles. The similarity between cognitive process of primitive people and immature children is the focal point. Werner provides a wealth of evidence from across the different regions of the world in support of his theory of mental development. Both the primitive people and immature children show diffused indifferentiated thinking, animism, magical thinking concretism. In contrast, civilized people and mature children show articulation, organized abstract thinking. Even in this approach, stages are not totally excluded. The development is regarded as a progress in an orderly and specifiable fashion from a state of relative generality to a stage of increasing differentiation. The arguments concerning the pattern of cognitive development, as mentioned, have made a deep impact on research studies, specially dealing with cultural factors involved.

Piaget (1963) and his co-workers have formulated what is considered to be the most systematic and comprehensive theory of cognitive growth based on naturalistic and scientific observational studies. Central to this theory is the convincing empirical evidence to establish "stage dependent invariant order of development". It is presumed that there is an active process where perceptual experience (Categories) represents the general manner in which they are related as a result of interaction between the children and the external world. In the beginning, these representations are in the form of simple structures and gradually get transformed through assimilation and accommodation, and to more complex structures. This is a process of an orderly sequence of stages. It is admitted, that though invariant, this order or sequence may be accelerated or slow down, due to social and cultural influences, but the sequence itself remains unalterable. As can be seen, this theory is a biologically oriented and deals with the development as coming to terms with environment in terms of the ability to cope with it. The sequence of cognitive development is described as follows.

1. Sensori motor stage—birth to 2 or 3 years.
2. Pre operational thinking—2 or 3 to 7 or 8 years.
3. Concrete operation—7 or 8 to 11 or 12 years.
4. Formal operation—11 or 12 to 14 or 15 years.

Piaget conceptualizes different levels of cognitive development in terms of differences in the qualitative nature of cognitive process and emergence of new ones. Even though a new stage emerges at certain points in cognitive growth there is a continuity in the sequence of changes with certain unique structural characteristics at each stage. It is very important for any one dealing with children to identify these unique characteristics at each level, so that the children can be effectively managed.

Brunner (1966) approaches the studies in cognitive growth in a slightly different manner from that of piaget. Though he speaks of progress through qualitatively different stages, he distinguishes three main levels of processing information. He calls them inactive, iconic and the symbolic. In the enactive stage, the child acquires the capacity to move around to grasp etc., which helps the child in understanding space at this stage. At the iconic stage the child understands the world in terms of percepts and images of a concrete kind. However, the child is unable to relate this to one another. The third stage namely, symbolic, is a more general and abstract concept of the world in terms of words, numbers and ideas. There is conservation phenomena. Bruner's description of cognitive growth has brought clarity to our understanding of children growing up in backworld societies. It is familiar that children living in backward societies learn more through doing than through words, they imitate older children and adults and thus form concepts of the world around them.

Witkin's (1967) theory of field dependence/independence is relevant to the study of culture and perception because he believes that there is a normal course of cognitive development from the global end of the spectrum to the articulated end (Compare Werner, 1961). The young child does not clearly differentiate himself from his environment, but as he grows he becomes aware of the boundaries of his body and personality and gains a sense of separate identity. This process of psychological differentiation is reflected in his cognitive and perceptual styles.

Vernon (1970) has brought greater clarity into the intricate problem of cultural environment and cognitive and intellectual growth. He has explored the role of environment and other factors which hinder the development of abilities within the under-developed countries or minority groups. As a preliminary to this very influential work, he has redefined the cognitive ability by identifying three different meanings associated with the term. He speaks of intelligence A, B and C emphasizing the genetic foundation, the cumulative effects of the interaction with the environment and the measured ability of a child on a standard test. In comparing different cultural groups one has to give appropriate consideration to each one of this type. Vernon has gathered evidence by extensive surveys and environmental studies on the relationship between environmental influence and growth of cognitive and intellectual ability. It is reported that differences between type B and C as mentioned within a cultural group are largely genetically determined. However, when environmental differences are more extreme, their effects become very prominent. Some major environmental factors which have a positive influence on mental development are:

1. Nutritional and health conditions.
2. Perceptual and sensori-motor experiences.

3. Language.
4. Child rearing practices and parental attitudes.

Jensen (1973) has put forward what is considered as a novel conception that environment affects development mainly as a "threshold variable". He argues that environment operates like diet in relation to physical growth. This kind of argument has aroused a great deal of controversy in the area of cultural differences in the growth of abilities. Jensen has shown that conventional tests of intelligence probably give better indications of all-round learning ability in middle class children than in lower class children. He speaks of two types of abilities namely, associated ability and cognitive ability which are independent in so far as they underline genetic aspects. The former measures the breadth aspect of ability while the latter describes the attitude aspects of the ability. In terms of the function, information and vocabulary are related to the breadth, problem solving and reasoning are related to the attitude, what is affected by environment and training is the breadth aspect of the ability. One of the most significant aspects of this approach is the relationship between socio-cultural aspects and intelligence. Jensen, expresses himself in favour of a largely genetic explanation of the evidence on racial and social group differences in educational performance. He certainly does not favour the orthodox view that all behavioural variation between groups is due to cultural differences, social discrimination and inequalities of opportunity.

Cognition which refers to the higher processes involved in understanding and dealing with the world around us is the foundation on which all the educational experiences of the child have to be built (Kuppuswamy, 1976). Cognitive process are especially important in such complex kinds of learning in remembering, forming concept, learning to solve problems and applying learned information to new situation (Sorenson, et al., 1975).

The cognitive correlates of creativity have been found to be divergent thinking abilities and some other abilities from convergent, cognition and evaluation categories. The more significant among them are those of transformation, implications and systems of product parameters. Similarly, other such abilities are involved in problem solving.

Creativity may be thought of as a quality or talent leading to a result which is novel and useful. The process involves interplay among a person, a task and social environment. Creativity springs from innermost recesses of human vision. It has been recognised as a precious source of emergence, development and survival of man's culture through ages.

Creativity has been viewed as a normally distributed trait, an aptitude trait, an intrapsychic-process, and as a style of life. It has been described as related to or one that can be equated with productivity, positive mental health and originality.

THEORETICAL BACKGROUND OF CREATIVITY

Psycho-dynamics of Thinking

A fundamental distinction within the psychoanalytic theory of thinking is that between primary process thinking, which is impulse driven and largely irrational, seeking immediate gratification at all costs even by way of hallucinations and secondary process thinking, which is logical and willing to postpone gratification for future gains. Kris (1952) stressed the importance for creativity of "regression in the service of ego" by which the freedom of primary process thinking was utilized for assembling the fantasy material that could, then he sorted out and refined by way of secondary process thinking. A similar idea was employed by Koestler (1964) who has given one of the more intelligible and respectable discussions of creative thinking.

Creativity may be regarded as the function of environmental factors and the personality of the individual child. Writers on psycho-analysis often stress the relevance of genetic (developmental) as well as a dynamic theory (Hartmann and Kris, 1945). This theory suggests that the influences to which the young child is susceptible unusually will leave a permanent mark on his creativity. While the problems have not been formulated clearly in terms of learning i.e., why and in what manner the results of childhood learning are more permanent than later learning. There are some kind of evidence supporting the gross facts of consequences in adulthood of early childhood experiences (Wolf, 1941; Beach and Jaynes, 1954; Whiting and Child, 1953 and Nijhawan, 1971).

Gowan's (1967) Theories Of Creativity

Creativity As Sound Mental Health

This view of creativity, which owes a great deal to Maslow, sees creativity in terms of complete character integration or lack of barriers between the conscious mind and it's preconscious areas.

While it is incumbent upon the child to develop emergent synthesizing abilities at higher actualizing levels, it is binding upon society to see that his prior need are satisfied to the extent that he can denote his energies to intellectual tasks. The child who is insecure about love and safety needs is too preoccupied to apply himself/herself.

Function of The Child's Oedipal Response to the Affectional Approach of the Opposite Sexed Parent

According to this theory, during the period from four to seven, the child enhanced by the warm affection of the opposite sexed parent responds to this in the only way he can by the creative manipulation of his immediate environment, and by an enlargement of the bridge between his fantasy life and his real world.

The Opposite Of Authoritarianism

This theory visualizes that the compartmentalization, stereotyping and anti-interception of the authoritarian personality prevents creative functioning. Hence, the degree to which we have been ramished with authoritarian practice diminishes our creative potential and narrows the possible avenues of creative endeavour. This view of creativity suggests that children can be helped to preserve their creativity by non-authoritarian attitudes on the part of parents and teachers, especially by not having negative evaluations put upon their initial efforts.

Piaget's (1967) Theory

The central assumption in Piaget (1967) analysis of cognitive change is his belief that development depends upon a continuous interaction between organism and environment—an interaction which involves, on one hand, environmental forces (people, objects, events) acting upon the child and on the other hand, the child acting selectively upon the environment. Piaget thinks "the human being is immersed right from birth in a social environment, which affects him just as the physical environment". Society, even more in a sense than physical environment, changes the very structure of the individual because it not only compels him to recognize the facts, but provides him with a ready-made system of signs and it imposes on him an infinite series of obligations. It is, there fore, quite evident that social life may affect creativity as it affects intelligence through the three media of language (Sign), content of interaction (values), and rules imposed on thought (collective logical and prelogical).

The mechanism of intellectual progress, Piaget believes, consists of assimilation. This is, reality data (environmental stimuli) are modified to enable them to be incorporated into existing structures. Piaget sees the adaptive interaction between organism and environment as involving the complementary processes of assimilation and accommodation. Assimilation names the process whereby the organism utilizes something from the environment and incorporates it.

Like Piaget (1971), Bruner (1962) also views creativity as a vital aspect of general intellectual development. Their cognitive developmental views focus on the recording of previously unrelated elements (Feldman, (1973) . Creativity is associated with moving from one stage of cognitive development to another, restoring equilibrium by reorganizing previously unrelated element through a new set of rules. The new stage is more stable, inclusive and encompassing than the previous one (Flawell, 1963).

Other Theories

Creativity has been considered to be one of the highest attainments of the human intellect. It is manifested in a variety of forms at various levels. Rogers (1962) insist on a tangible product, such as a poem, a work of art or scientific theory. Stein (1953) calls the process as creative when it results in "novel work that is acceptable as tenable or useful or satisfying by a group at some point in time."

Guiford's (1962) theory of creativity says that a creative person is not necessarily creative all round but is capable of creativity in certain specific areas and not in others.

Mednic (1962) has advanced a theory of creativity which is of the associative sort. He suggests that divergent people tend to link stimuli with highly unlikely responses, whereas in most people any particular stimulus is usually linked with the response with which it has most frequently been paired in the past.

THE SCOPE AND IMPORTANCE OF THE PRESENT STUDY

Creativity is the ultimate answer to man's problems, innovation of new ideas and things and ultimately the civilization of life. The value and worth of this potential is unlimited. The future of our nation depends upon the creative talents of the future citizens of society. Therefore, creativity has become a chief psycho-social motive of the twentieth century. Creativity is a kind of psychic wonder (Singh, 1977).

Creativity is a unique gift of nature, a highly valued human quality which has been known for a long time to have it's influence on scientific, technological and artistic spheres of human activity. The rapidly changing demands and challenges existing in the world today have almost necessarily been accompanied by creative expression and contributions from talented persons. When we look critically at the present day educational practice, one of the lacunae is a lack of importance given to creativity. Singh (1977), Watsa (1979) and Sumangala (1987) reported that the Indian educational system is failing to develop children's latent abilities and intelligence and therefore, also failing to prepare them for rational and creative living. This being so, it is necessary to generate research data on creativity and performance when excellence is given the highest premium.

The performance and attainment of a child in the present educational system depends very much upon perceptual growth and efficient cognitive styles. Cognitive style is a psychological construct which contains elements of perceptual styles, personality, intelligence and social behaviour. Cognitive styles have been linked to many areas of problem-solving, academic achievement and socio-emotional behaviour. To understand how cognitive styles influence academic achievements, well carried out research is needed.

Singer and Rummo (1973) suggested that creativity may be related to the "possession of a free-wheeling cognitive style". Duffy (1978) found cognitive style to be a good predictor of creativity. At a more general level Kogan (1973) noticed that the similarity of processes underlying both creativity and cognitive style has encouraged research in this area.

It is presumed that progress in varied dimensions like economic growth, technological development and psychological well-being of person becomes possible through the creative talents and appropriate cognitive style.

Though everyone has creative ability to some extent and tend to use one or the other cognitive styles, some one may be more fortunate to realize his own potentialities in greater measure. It is perhaps true that most of the tribal children in India who are in a way disadvantaged may not seem to get fair opportunities to foster better growth in contrast to their counterparts who are better placed in the society. As a result, the cognitive development of these disadvantaged children, particularly creativity and cognitive styles may not reach optimal level.

The general factors that are influencing creativity and cognitive styles are demographic, psychological and environmental.

The review presented in the second chapter of the study clearly reveals that there is interrelationship between creativity and cognitive styles (Soptts and Mackler, 1967; Kaufman, 1975; Noppe, 1977; Smilansky and Halberstadt, 1986; Fuque, Bartsch and Phye, 1975 and Klein, Blockovich, Buchalter and Huyhe, 1976). All these studies were conducted in western context but the studies in Indian context appear to be meagre and studies attempting to examine the interrelation between creativity and cognitive styles are more needed.

Similarly, a few studies were conducted on influence of demographic factors like ethnicity and creativity and cognitive styles (Bhan 1970; Hurlock, 1981; Richmond, 1971; Halpin, Halpin and Torrance. 1973; Raina, 1968; Badarinadh and Sathyanarayana, 1979; Chandha and Sen, 1981; Venkata Rami Reddy and Tulsi Devi, 1981; Ahmed and Joshi, 1978; Ahmed, 1980; Krishna Kumari, Lalitha and Paramaji, 1986; Golwalker, 1986; Sharma, 1972; Okonji, 1969; Smith, 1971; Marjoribanks, 1978; Tharakan, 1987; Dash and Dash, 1980; and Smith and Ribordy, 1980) by Western and Indian researchers. But the results are not conclusive. With regard to age and creativity, a few studies have been available in western and Indian culture (Piers, et al., 1960; Olshin, 1965; Trowbridge and Charles, 1966; Passi, 1972; Paramesh, 1970; Ahmed, 1980; Joshi, 1974; Gakhar, 1975; Dharmangadan, 1981; Venkata Rami Reddy and Balakrishna Reddy, 1988; Raina, 1970) which shows inconsistent results. Similarly, the results of sex differences and creativity are varied and not conclusive (Straus and Straus, 1968; Mar I, 1971; Raina, 1969; Rawat and Agarwal, 1977; Tara, 1981; Dharmangadan, 1981; Bhaskara, 1986; Torrance, 1967; Orcutt, 1968; Torrance and Aliotti, 1969; Macgregor and Smith, 1965; Ogletree, 1968; Solomen, 1968; Walker, 1969; Cacha, 1971; Burgess, 1971; Kershner and Ledger, 1985; Hussain, 1974; Singh, 1978; Raina, 1980; Chandha and Ghose, 1985; Asifa, 1987; Maccoby and Jacklin, 1974; Ward and Cox, 1974; Phatak, 1962; Jackson, 1968; Simpkins and Eisenman, 1968; Burns, 1969; Kaltsounis, 1971; Phillips and Torrance,

1971; Kloss, 1972; Jarial, 1982; and Venkateswara Rao, 1987). Only a few western studies are reported on age and sex differences and cognitive styles (Crandall and Sinkeldam, 1964; Witking, Goodenough and Karp, 1967; Coates, 1971; Kogan, 1976; Huss and Kayson, 1985; Drouin, Talbot and Goulet, 1986; Bill, 1987; Ault, 1973; Campbell and Douglas, 1972; Fancher, 1969; Kayan, 1965; Ward, 1973; Wright, 1973; and Salkind and Wight, 1977). But the investigator has not come across any Indian studies. To know more concretely how these factors influence the creativity and cognitive styles in tribal and non-tribal children, a more specific research is needed in the Indian context.

The research data generated on the influence of psychological factors like personality and creativity (Parloff and Datta, 1966; Kurtzman, 1967; Iwata, 1968; White, 1968; Khire, 1971; Komarik, 1972; Hassan and Akbar, 1973; Phillips, 1973; Wolters, 1976; Goyal, 1969; Ahmad, 1969; Passi, 1972; Paramesh, 1972; Gakhar, 1975; Passi and Lalitha, 1975; Nair, 1975; Jawa, 1976; Patel, 1976; Paramesh and Narayana, 1976; Babu, 1977; Chauhan, 1977; Mehdi, 1977; Mallapa and Upadhyaya, 1977; Kumar, 1978; Asha, 1978; Bhattacharya, 1978; Singh, 1978; Jhag, 1979; Jairal and Sharma, 1980; Muddu, 1980; Gakhar and Joshi, 1980; Kishore, 1981; Chandha and Sen, 1981; Agarwal and Bohra, 1982; Goyal, 1984; Helode, 1986; Matthews, 1986; Kundu, 1986; and Kumar and Kumari, 1988) were many in western and Indian context. But the results are equivocal and inconsistent. With regard to research on personality and cognitive styles (Goodenough and Karp, 1961; Vaught, 1965; Kato, 1965; Pederson and Wender, 1968; Vernon, 1972; Goodenough, 1976; Panek, 1982; Goodenough, Oltman and Cox, 1987; Kagan, and Kogan, 1970; Messer, 1970; Thomas, 1971; Kagan, 1965; Finch, Pezzuti Montgomery and Kemp, 1974; Block, et al., 1974; Bannigan and Ash, 1977; Messer and Brosdzinsky, 1979; Finch and Kendall, 1979; Wiedl and Bathge, 1981; Victor, Halverson and Montague, 1985; and Lajoie and Shore, 1987) was considerable in Western countries but not in India. Very few studies seem to be reported in Western and Indian cultures on locus of control and creativity and cognitive styles (Davis and Phares, 1967; Brecher and Denmark, 1969; Bolen and Torrance, 1978; Richmond and serna, 1980; Agarwal and Verma, 1977; Crandall and Lacey, 1972; Davis, 1982; Max, Howard and Winne, 1987; Tripathi and Tripathi, 1984; Shipe, 1971; Messer, 1972; Berzonsky, 1974 and Massari, 1975). Hence, the present study is an attempt to know the influence of psychological (personality and locus of control factors on creativity and cognitive styles in tribal and non-tribal children.

Some research studies in western countries and a very few studies in India were conducted on the influence of environmental factors like home environment and creativity and cognitive styles (Watson, 1957; Roe, 1960; Orienstein, 1961; Weisberg and Springer, 1961; Singer, 1961; Getzels and Jackson, 1962; Mackinnon 1962; Stein, 1963; Nichols, 1964; Dyk and Witkin, 1965; Dryer and Wells, 1966; Nuttal, 1969; Silverberg, 1970; Eisenman and Foxman, 1970; Wade, 1971; Walberg, 1971; Swan and Stavra, 1973; Dewing, 1973; Aldous, 1975; Moore and Bulbulian, 1976; Shmukler, 1982-83; Fu, Moran, Sawters and Milgram, 1983; Sinha and Sharma, 1978; Dyk and Witkin, 1965; Barclay and Cusumano, 1967; Goldstein and Peak, 1973; Witkin and Berry, 1975; Kagan and Lawrence, 1982; and Paul, 1986). But the results of these studies are not conclusive. Therefore, it is necessary to focus in these direction to know the influence of environmental factor (home environment) on creativity and cognitive styles of tribal and non-tribal children.

The above discussion clearly reveals the need for comprehensive attempt to generate data on scientific lines which throw light on the nature of creativity and cognitive styles and their relationship, the influence of factors like demographic (ethnicity, age and sex), psychological (personality and locus of control) and environmental (home environment) on creativity and cognitive styles. The present study is focusing on the above lines to understand the development aspects of children as to take corrective measures by the teachers, parents and community.

THE RESEARCH PROBLEM

"A study of certain factors influencing creativity and cognitive styles in tribal and non-tribal children."

The following are the research questions framed for the study:

1. Is there a significant relationship between creativity and cognitive styles?
2. In what way and how some of the important demographic (ethnicity, age and sex), psychological (personality and locus of control) and environmental (home environment) factors influence the expression of creativity and cognitive styles?

3. Is there a differential incidence of verbal and non-verbal components of creativity among the tribal and non-tribal children?
4. Out of the two cognitive styles (field dependence/independence and reflection/impulsivity), which cognitive style is predominantly seen in tribal and non-tribal children?

TERMS USED IN THE STUDY

Tribe

India has the largest tribal (ethnic group) population compared to any other single country in the world. There are more than 427 tribal communities in India. According to the recommendations of the Indian Constitution almost all the tribal communities are considered scheduled tribes.

Tribe is derived from the Latin word *tribus* meaning "one-third" which originally referred to one of the three territorial groups that united to found Rome. The Romans later applied tribus to the 35 people who became a part of Rome before 241 B.C still later the Romans applied the term tribus to segments of the Gallic or Germanic populations whom they conquered.

The word tribe means a hoard of people bound together by definite relations, social, moral, aesthetic, intellectual and of all other kinds that are possible. In other words tribe is a strictly homogeneous unit of members who constitute it.

More widely used definition of tribe is a collection of families or groups of families bearing a common name, members of which occupy the same territory, speak the same language and observe certain taboos regarding marriage, profession or occupation and have developed a well assessed system of reciprocity and mutually of obligations (Majumdar, 1950).

Bailey (1961) offered the following criteria to explain the features of a tribe:

1. *Geographical isolation*: Each tribe occupies a particular geo-graphical area. One has little communication with the outside world.
2. *Language*: By and large each tribe has it's own language.

3. *Religion*: Tribals are animists.
4. *Economy*: They are usually economically backward, they live mostly by primitive techniques.
5. *Nativity and origin*: They are literally adivasis or autochthones.
6. *Heterogeneity of occupation*; They do not have specific occupations.

Characteristics Of Tribal Societies

Some of the following characteristics are commonly, though not universally found in tribal societies.

1. It has longer history than any other type of society.
2. It is a whole society. All the needs and services required by a community are normally fulfilled by that tribal society.
3. It has special feature of normative structure which binds together the members of the society.
4. The culture of tribal society is the culture of silence.
5. Tribals have their own specific eco-system.
6. Tribals practice polygyny as an institution of prestige and glory.
7. Tribal society is homogeneous.
8. It is largely based on clan system.
9. It is autonomous and has a strong self-perpetuating political organization.
10. It most commonly remains in a common territory, has a common name, speaks a common language, shares a common culture, practices endogamy and possesses a sense of mutual unity among it's members.
11. Tribal society is one which is heavily addicted to liquor drinking.

It is worth mentioning that tribal characteristics are not rigid in the Indian social structural context. Ghurye (1957) did not totally agree with the view that the tribal characteristics are strictly tribal in nature.

After the attainment of independence in 1947, the Government of India has been making consistent effort to bring the tribal population into the mainstream of society. The state Government of Andhra Pradesh like the other states also started colonizing the tribals and inspiring them to become settled agriculturists. But, occupational structures of tribals often change depending on their survival needs. However, the traditional tribes have been influenced by the Government welfare measures as well as urbanization and industrialization with the result that they are in a state of transition at present.

Ghurye (1957) called the tribes as "Backward Hindus" which suggests that they are among the Hindu castes. Sachidananda, Firma and Mukhopadhyay (1965), believe that the tribes have acquired the characteristics of a caste although they keep the tribal culture intact.

Non-Tribe

The definition of a caste or non-tribe is a hereditary endogamous, usually localized group having traditional association with an occupation and a particular position in the local hierarchy of castes. Relations between castes are governed, among other things by the concepts of pollution and purity, and generally maximum commensality occurs within the caste (Srinivas, 1962).

Writers on caste or non-tribal such as Hutton (1963), Ketkar (1903), Ghurye (1957), Srinivas (1962) and others have agreed on the basic attributes of the non-tribe which are as follows:

1. Endogamy.
2. Membership by birth.
3. Occupational specialization.
4. An ideological religious basis involving restrictions on social intercourse and commensality.
5. Co-operativeness of the group at least on a local level.
6. It directs it's economic behaviour in terms of deferred gratification.
7. It is linked with peasant society.
8. It welcomes a change.

Characteristics Of Non-Tribal Societies

As peasant and urban societies come under non-tribal societies, their characteristics are given as follows:

Peasant Society

1. It has long history commensurate with that of city and state.
2. It has a social system based on face-to-face relationships.
3. It views agriculture as a means of livelihood not as a business for profit.
4. It is based on antiquated technology and low agricultural productivity.
5. It directs it's economic behaviour at a pattern of immediate consumption and at meeting the material demands of ceremonialism.
6. It always maintains communication with the urban centres;
7. It is resistant or very slow to change.

Urban Society

1. It has extended history parallel to that of a peasant society. The urban and peasant society are twins, they are born simultaneously.
2. It is heterogeneous.
3. It has frequent travel and communication in and with the larger society.
4. It has a social system based on highly impersonal relations.
5. It has an economic system based on a complex division of labour and production for trade.

Creativity

The standard definition of creativity is becoming sensitive to or aware of problems, deficiencies, gaps in knowledge, missing elements, disharmonies and so on; bringing together available information; defining the difficulty or identifying the missing element; searching for solutions, making guesses or formulating hypotheses about the deficiencies, testing and retesting these hypotheses and modifying and restating them; perfecting them and finally communicating the results (Torrance, 1962).

Concept of Creativity

According to Mathur and George (1985) creativity has become delineated into a number of aspects like dimensionality, dynamics, personality and measurement.

Sharma and Sharma (1987) remark that the use of creativity by educators and psychologists is highly individualistic. Malhara (1985) points out that creativity has two aspects : one, the process of creation and two, the product of creation. While the process of creation is an inner happening, the products of creativity can be seen and defined.

Components of Creativity

The concepts of imagination, fantasy, fluency, flexibility, originality, elaboration, curiosity and giftedness have been studied in children and in many cases have been equated with creativity.

Imagination

Andrews (1930) has defined imagination in children as "the process by which items of experience are combined to form new products".

Fantasy

The terms "imagination" and "fantasy" have been used interchangeably. Both Griffiths (1945) and Singer (1961) equate fantasy with day dreams and imaginative play and the resulting images thereby produced; the term "imagination" is more often used to describe the process rather than the product.

Fluency

It means the frequency with which relevant and unrepeated ideas come to one's mind after a question is put.

Flexibility

It is represented by a person's ability to produce ideas which differ in approval or thought trend.

Originality

It is uniqueness of response. Guilford (1962) defines originality as "the production of unusual, for fetched, remote or clever responses among members of a certain population that is culturally homogeneous".

Elaboration

It is indicated by a person's ability to add pertinent details (more ideas) to the minimum and primary response to the stimulus figure

Curiosity

Medinnus and love (1965) define curiosity in terms of exploratory behaviour and use four measures of curiosity; Peer and teacher's ratings, object curiosity, preference for an unknown toy and preference for a story - ending devoting the satisfaction of curiosity.

Giftedness

Terman's (1959) original study of giftedness in children was primarily based on I Q measures, but his 25-year and 35-year follow-up studies (Terman, 1947, 1959) revealed that, on the basis of childhood I Qs, about 20 per cent of the men did not attain the level of achievement he had predicted. After examining their family and childhood environment, he concluded that "personality factors are extremely important determinants of achievement".

Until recently, only the child with a high IQ was considered gifted, but a distinction is now made between such aspect of giftedness (or talent) as intelligence, musical and artistic ability, creative writing, and even social leadership (Burt, 1962; Witty, 1962).

Among all these components, primary ones are fluency, flexibility, originality and elaboration and these appear to operate creative thinking of children and these are studied in present investigation.

Cognitive Styles

Cognitive process refers to all the processes by which the sensory input is transformed, reduced, elaborated, stored and used. The concern is with how the individual gets, creates, and uses knowledge about physical and social world. Until last decade, individual difference in the cognitive processes of perception, memory and problem solving were viewed as reflecting difference in basic intelligence, anxiety, conflict attitudes to these individual differences has been explored.

Pattern of thought and behaviour that influence learning and problem - solving techniques are known as "cognitive styles". A cognitive style is an individual "manner and form of cognitive performance" (Siegel and Brodzinky, 1977) and reflects that individuals's personality or performance, not his or her ability or intelligence.

Cognitive styles refers to the different modes of functioning that characterize an individual's perceptual and intellectual faculties (Witkin, et al., 1967). They are dimensional in the expression.

Theorists have studied the development aspects of three major cognitive styles namely field dependence/independence, reflection/ impulsivity and categorization styles. These constitute a set of three established properties of the behavior of perceptual responses system (Kagan, 1966) The brief account of these is as follows:

Field Dependence/independence

It has been defined by Witkin, et al (1954) in terms of the capacity of overcome embedding contexts in perception. Subjects who readily accept the prevailing field or context who have difficulty in separating an item from it's context are called field dependent; subjects who easily "break-up" an organized perceptual field - who can readily separate an item from it's context are called field independent.

It refers to variations in people's perceptual cognitive perspectives of their experience. The field independent person tends to experience his surroundings analytically, with objects experienced as discrete from their backgrounds. The field dependent person, on the other hand, perceives his surroundings in a relatively global fashion, with objects confirming to or indistinguishable from the background (Witkin, Dyk, Faterson, Goodenough and Karp, 1962). Patterns of child rearing have been cited as one of the possible origins of field dependence/independence (Dyk and Witkin, 1965).

Compared with field dependent subjects, field independent subjects perceive the following; (1) more readily disembodied a simple figure which has emerged in a complex design, (2) more accurately adjust their seated bodies to an upright position in a tilted room, (3) more accurately adjust to an upright position on luminous rod which is surrounded by tilted square frame, and (4) draw human figures in a more articulated fashion. What underlies each of these tendencies is an ability to deal with a part of a field separately from the field as a whole. Whereas field dependent persons tend to structure their experience by using external referents, field independent subjects use internal referents. In estimating time, field dependent persons to use available referents in the prevailing field.

Individuals respond to different situations based on their particular cognitive style. Characteristics of cognitive styles have been consistent and stable. Field dependent individuals rely on authority figures and are sensitive to the feelings of others, as expressed in social skills. Field independent individuals are oriented towards active striving and are socially detached, possessing analytic skills.

Reflection/impulsivity

The definition of reflection/impulsivity cognitive style is a conceptual tempo or decision time variable, representing the time the subject takes consider alternative solutions before committing himself to one of them in situation with high response uncertainty .

It measures the degree to which an individual evaluates possible response alternatives in situations of moderate to high response uncertainty. Children who take their time before offering a response and who subsequently produce few errors have been termed reflective, while children who are quick and inaccurate in their initial responding have been termed impulsive. Two additional groups of children (show-inaccurates and fast-accurate) are also categorized (Block, Block and Harrington, 1974; Kagan and Kogan, 1970; Messer, 1970). The origin of the reflection-impulsivity style is unknown.

Compared with reflective individuals impulsive appear to (1) have problems in delaying gratifications, (2) made quick decisions, (3) show less persistence at tasks and (4) become more easily bored; preter novel or unpredictable stimuli. One possible explanation for each of these four characteristics processed by impulsive persons is a distorted perception of time.

The reflective child is viewed as less likely than the impulsive child to report wrong solution; more likely to consider alternative possibilities before committing himself; preferring low-risk situations generally but choosing harder, more solitary intellectual tasks; having a longer attention span; and being less distractible, less motorically active and more cautious than impulsive age mates.

Categorization Styles

These are the types of groupings by means of which a person

classifies or arranges stimuli. Several people presented with the same objects will justify grouping them according to different criteria. Categorization style have been sub divided into three types. A descriptive analytic style concentrates on a single obvious detail common to all the objects ("they are all straight"). The relational - contextual approach seizes on a common theme or function. ("They are all used to connect two objects"). A categorical - inferential style focuses on the class of the object (tools, fasteners, studs, etc.).

Among the three cognitive styles, only two (field dependence/independence, reflection/impulsivity) styles are well recognised. In the present study, the cognitive style refers to field dependence/independence, reflection/impulsivity.

Certain Factors

Demographic Factors

In this study, demographic factors include ethnicity, age and sex of the Sugali tribal and non-tribal children.

Psychological Factors

Personality

Personality is the organisation of an individuals distinguishing characteristics, attitudes or habits; it includes the individuals unique ways of thinking, behaving or otherwise experiencing the environment (Benjamin, Hopkins, Nation, 1987).

The configuration of characteristics and behaviour that comprises an individuals unique adjustment to life, including major traits, interests, drives, values, self-concept, abilities and emotional patterns. Personality is generally viewed as complex dynamic integration of totality shaped by many forces; heredity and constitutional tendencies, physical maturation, early training, identification with significant individuals and groups, culturally conditioned values and roles and critical experiences and relationships.

Personality is shaped by in-born potential as modified by experiences common to culture, such as the various roles the individual is called upon to play and by the unique experience that affect him as an individual.

Locus of Control

Locus of control is a generalized expectancy concerning the

relationship, between behaviour and outcome. Interpretation of events as contingent upon ones own actions reflects as internal locus of control and those perceived as independent of ones behaviour reflect a belief in external locus of control (Rotter, 1966).

The construct of locus of control as outlined by Rotter (1966) has been used to predict a wide range of behaviour. It is a concept which developed from the domain of social learning theory (Rotter, 1964 and Rotter, Chance and Pyhares, 1972) in which expectations regarding the probability of reinforcement are hypothesized to be important determinants of behaviour. Rotter (1966) subsequently proposed that differences in such expectations are due in part to an enduring personality trait, which has become known as locus of control. Persons believing that they control over the likelihood of experiencing reinforcing outcomes are referred to as internally - to chance, fate, luck, or powerful others - are termed externals. Obviously, most people fall between the two extremes, forming a continuous distribution of locus of control beliefs. Locus of control is thought to be relatively enduring dispositional characteristic, although certainly modifiable through experience.

Locus of control is a cognitive personality construct that has been found to be related to many important dimensions of human functioning (Lefcourt, 1966).

Environmental Factor

Home Environment

Home environment is a measure of the quality and quantity of social, emotional and cognitive support that has been available to the child within the home (Misra, 1986). The most important part of the child's environment is the home. Family is the society in miniature and the child is in the home and the home alone for the first vital years of his life. When he starts going to school, he is there only for a part of his time (Young and McGreney, 1968). Home is the most important in child's life, because it is the home that meets the child's basic needs whether they are physical, psychological, social and emotional. Sagar and Kaplan (1972) pointed out, by its nature, the family is the social, biological unit that exerts the greatest influence on the development and perpetuation of the individuals behaviour.

The term "home environment" as such or as a synonym of

parental child-rearing behaviours have been used by many re-searchers wording in different fields. According to Johnson and Medinnus (1969), the psychological atmosphere of a home may fall into any of the four quadrants, each of which represents one of the four general combinations: acceptance - autonomy, acceptance-control, rejection-autonomy, and rejection-control.

Acceptance
(Love)

Autonomy --------------- Control
(Democratic) (Autocratic)

Rejection
(Hostility)

Two characteristics occur throughout the studies of Symonds (1939), Baldwin, Kalhorn and Breese (1945) and Lorr and Jenkins (1953). These are acceptance versus, rejection and autonomy versus control. Grebow (1973) reports that the dimensions of parental behaviour which have been most consistently suggested as important by previous research are a) nurturance - affection and b) achievement expectations, demands and standards (Crandall, Preston and Rabson, 1960; Crandall, Katkovsky and Preston, 1960; Gandall, Dewey, Katkovsky and Perston, 1964; Rosen and D'Andrade, 1959 and Winterbottom, 1958).

The review of related literature of the present study has been reported in the next chapter.

2

REVIEW OF RELATED LITERATURE

In this chapter an attempt is made to present a survey of the review of literature related to the research topic. The following scheme of classification was evolved to make the presentation more, methodical and meaningful.

Contributions to the Measurement of Creativity and Cognitive Styles

Contributions to the measurement of creativity.

Contributions to the measurement of field dependence/independence cognitive style.

Contributions to the measurement of reflection/impulsivity cognitive style.

Studies on Inter-relation between creativity and Cognitive Styles

Studies on inter-relation between creativity and fields dependence/independence cognitive style.

Studies on inter-relation between creativity and reflection/impulsivity cognitive style.

Influence of Demographic Factors on Creativity and Cognitive Styles

Studies on ethnicity and creativity.

Studies on ethnicity and field dependence/independence cogni-

tive style.

Studies on ethnicity and reflection/impulsivity cognitive style.

Studies on age and creativity.

Studies on sex differences and creativity.

Studies on age and sex difference and field dependence/independence cognitive style.

Studies on age and sex differences and reflection/impulsivity cognitive style.

Influence of Psychological Factors on Creativity and Cognitive Styles

Studies on personality and creativity.

Studies on personality and field dependence/independence cognitive style.

Studies on personality and reflection/impulsivity cognitive style.

Studies on locus of control and creativity.

Studies on locus of control and field dependence/independence cognitive style.

Studies on locus of control and reflection/impulsivity cognitive style.

Influence of Environment Factors on Creativity and Cognitive Styles

Studies on home environment and creativity.

Studies on home environment and field dependence/independence cognitive style.

CONTRIBUTIONS TO THE MEASUREMENT OF CREATIVITY AND COGNITIVE STYLE

Contributions to the Measurement of Creativity

As a result of the scientific and systematic studies in the field of creativity, many educators, psychologists directed their efforts to develop various tools for identifying creative individuals. A number of tests have emerged most important as developed by Guiford (1960), Mednick (1962), Getzels and Jackson (1962), Torrance widely and indiscriminately used. Various researchers in India have also made use of these tests.

Gulford's Contribution

In 1958 when the Bureau of Educational Research of the University of Minnesota began it's studies of creative thinking, it felt that what was needed was a set of tasks which could be used from kindergarten through graduate school. Thus, it first attempted to adapt Guiford's (1951) materials with this objective in mind.

The Bureau developed as a start two alternate forms of the following Guilford-type tasks: unusual uses, impossibilities, consequences, problem situations, improvements and problems.

Guilford had hypothesized that the thinking abilities involved in creativity were those he had defined as divergent productions and transformations. He included the redefinition abilities which were in the convergent - production category of his structure of intellect and sensitivity to problems which fill in the evaluation category. Thus, the following factors and tasks for assessing them may be regarded as summarizing Guilford's present theory concerning measurement of the thinking abilities involved in creativity (Guilford and Merrifield, 1960).

Factor	Tests and Descriptions
Sensitivity to problems (Seeing defects; needs; deficiencies; seeing the odd; the unusual; seeing what must be done).	Apparatus Test—suggests two improvements for a common appliance.
	Seeing Problems—list of problems that might arise in connection with common objects.
	Seeing Deficiencies—point out the way in which a described plan or activity is fault.
Figural spontaneous flexibility	Cube Fluctuations—indicate the number of changes in perspective of ambiguous cube.
	Windmill/Alternations—indicate the number of alternations from the illusion to another while observing shadow of rotating rectangular blade.
	Retinal-rivalry Reversals—indicate the number of reversals when a blue field is presented stereoscopically to one eye and a yellow field to the other eye.

Contd.

Factor	Tests and Descriptions
Figural adaptive flexibility	Match Problems II—indicate three or four different patterns of a specified number of matches that can be removed to leave a specified number of triangles or squares. Match Problems III— indicate several different patterns of matches that can be removed to leave a specified number of squares. Planning air maneuvers select the most direct path is "sky-writing" letter combinations.
Word fluency	Suffixes W-1—write words ending with a specified suffix (ETS). Prefixes W-2—write words beginning with a specified prefix. First and last letters W-3-write words beginning and ending with a specified letter.
Expressional fluency	Write four-word sentences when the first letter of each word is given. Simile Interpretations—complete sentence that states an analogous idea. Word Arrangements—write sentences containing four specified words.
Ideational fluency	Topics if-1—write as many ideas as possible about a given topic. Then if-2—write as many words as possible about a given topic. Categories if-3—list the names of things that are round or that can be called round.
Semantic spontaneous flexibility	Brick Uses (flexibility)—write a variety of uses of a brick. Alternative Uses—list different peculiar uses for common objects.
Associational fluency	Controlled Associations—Write as many synonyms as possible for each given word. Simile Insertions—write adjectival completion for simile.

(Contd.)

Factor	Tests and Descriptions
	Associations IV—produce a word that can be associated with two given words. Associational fluency I—write synonyms for given words.
Originality	Plot Titles (clever)—write clever titles for story plots. Symbol production—produce symbols to represent activities and objects. Consequences (remote)—list remote consequences of certain changes.
Semantic elaboration	Planning Elaboration—fill in as many details as necessary to make a briefly outlined activity work. Figure Production—add to given lines to produce a meaningful figure score is based on number of details drawn.
Figural redefinition (defining or perceiving in a way different from the usual, established, or intended way, use etc.)	Concealed Figures CF-1—indicate which of your complex geometrical figures contains a given geometrical figure. Penetration of Camouflage—locate focus hidden in pictures. Hidden Pictures—find human or animal pictures hidden in a scene, as rapidly as possible. Hidden figures indicate which of five figures is hidden in a given figure.
Symbolic redefinition	Camouflaged Words—find the name of the sport or game concealed in a sentence. Word transformation indicate new divisions between letters in a new series of words forming a phrase, to make a new series of words.
Semantic redefinition	Gestalt Transformation—indicate which of five listed objects have a part that will serve a specified purpose. Object Synthesis—name an object that could be made by combining two specified objects. Picture Gestalt—indicate which object in a photograph will serve a specified purpose.

Mednick's Contribution

The Remote Association Test (RAT) was designed by Mednick (1962). In each item of these test, subjects are presented with three words which have some common association, and they are required to find a fourth word which has common associative links with all three stimulus words.

Getzels and Jackson's Contribution

Getzels and Jackson (1962) constructed 5 tests to measure creativity. They are (1) Word Association Test, (2) Uses Test, (3) Hidden Shape Test, (4) Fables Test, (5) Make-up Problems Test. They suggested two scoring procedures - one simple and the other elaborate. The correlation between the scores obtained in the two procedures was more than 0.90 for the different tests. The tests are briefly described as follows:

1. **Word Association Test:** This test presents the subjects with twenty five words, each of which has multiple meanings (e.g.: arm, cap, duck, fair etc.). The student is asked to write as many meanings as he can for each word.
2. **Uses Test:** It presents the subject with the names of five common objects (bricks, pencils, paper clips, tooth picks, sheet of paper) and asks him to write as many different uses by two examples - one representing a common use, the other an unusual use (e.g.: Brick - build houses, door stop).
3. **Hidden Shapes Test:** This test is part of Cattle's (1956) Objective Analytic Test battery and consists of eighteen simple geometric figures each of which is followed by four more complex figures. The subject's task is to identify the complex figures in which the simple figure appears.
4. **Fables Test :** It consists of four fables whose last lines are missing. The student is required to supply a moralistic, a humorous and a sad ending for each fable.
5. **Make-up Problems Test :** It consists of four complex paragraphs, each containing many numerical statements about activities such as buying a house, building a swimming pool, and the like. For each paragraph, the student is to use the information given to make up as many mathematical problems as he can within the limit. The single restriction is that the problems must

be capable of solution. The student must use only the material in the paragraph. The student is not required to solve problems.

Guilford's Test of Divergent Thinking, Mednick's Remote Association Test and Getzels and Jackson's Creativity indices were in use for sometime but these tests correlate quite high with the Torrance and Wallach and Kogan test and also are very comprehensive in their way to be in the field.

Torrance's Contribution

According to Arastech and Arashech (1976), the most systematic assessment of creativity in elementary school children has been conducted by Torrance and his associates (1960-1966) who have developed and administered the Minnesota Tests of Creative Thinking (MTC) to several thousand school children. Although they have used many of Guilford's concepts in their test construction, the Minnesota group, in contrast to Guilford, has devised tasks which can be scored for several factors, involving both verbal and non-verbal aspects and relying on senses other than vision.

Torrance (1962) grouped the MTCT into three categories: (1) Non-verbal tasks, (2) Verbal task using non-verbal stimuli, (3) Verbal tasks using verbal stimuli; Brief description of some of the tasks used by Torrance is given below.

(1) **Non-verbal Tasks:** Four non-verbal tasks have been used in the Minnesota studies.

Incomplete Figures Task: It is an adaptation of the Drawing Completion Test developed by Kate Frank and used in studies of creativity by Barron, et al (1958). On an ordinary sheet of paper an area of fifty-four square inches is divided into six squares, each containing a different stimulus figure. Subjects are given the following instructions concerning this task: By adding lines to the six figures, sketch some object or design that no one else in the class will think of. Try to include as many different ideas as you can in your drawing, don't stop with your first idea for completing the figure, keep building on to it. Make up titles for each of your pictures and write one at the bottom of each block next to the number of the figure. Before the subjects begin, the tests given them four examples for the first incomplete figure.

Responses to this task are evaluated along four different dimensions, originality, closure (penetration) complexity (elaboration) and productivity.

Picture-construction Task : In this task, subjects are required to think of a picture in which the given shape is an integral part. A blank sheet of paper and a piece of glued, coloured paper of a triangle and a curved jelly beam shape are given to the subjects with the following instructions: you have been given a piece of paper in the form of triangle (Curved shape). Think of a picture or an object which you can draw with this form as a part. Then lift up the shape and glue it wherever you want it on this sheet of paper and add lines with pencil or crayon to make your picture as many interesting ideas as you can. When you have completed your picture, think up a name or title for it and write it at the bottom. Responses are scored for originality, elaboration, sensitivity, communication and activity.

Circles and Squares Tasks : It was originally designed as a non verbal test of ideational fluency and flexibility, then modified in such a way as to stress originality and elaboration. Two printed forms are used in the test. On one of them thirty five (1" × 1") squares are printed and on the other, forty two small circles (1" diameter). Responses are scored for fluency, flexibility, originality and elaboration.

Creative Design Task : Hendrickson has designed it which seems to be promising, but scoring procedures are being tested but have not been perfected yet. The materials consist of circles and strips of various sizes and colours, a four-page booklet, scissors and glue. Subjects are instructed to the coloured circles and strips with a thirty-minute time limit. Subjects may use one, two, three, or four pages, alter the circles and strips or use them as they are, add other symbols with pencil or crayon.

(2) Verbal Tasks Using Non-verbal Stimuli

Ask and Guess Test: It requires the individual first to ask questions about a picture, questions which can not be answered by looking at the picture. Next he is asked to make guesses or formulate hypotheses about the possible causes and then the consequences, both immediate and remote of the behaviour depicted.

Responses can then be evaluated to yield scores on a number of Guiford factors such as, sensitivity to problems (number of missing piece-of-information questions were asked); ideational fluency (number of questions and guesses), flexibility (variety of kinds of questions and hypotheses) and originality.

Product Improvement Task : In this task common toys are used and children are asked to think of as many improvements as they can which would make the toy "more fun to play with". Subjects are then asked to think of unusual uses of these toys other than "something to play with". Responses are then scored for such factors as, fluency (number of improvements and unusual uses given), flexibility (number of approaches used in making improvements and number of categories of unusual uses), originality (number of uncommon improvements and uses), inventive level (a measure based on criteria used by the United States Patent Office in evaluating patent applications and meaning level of degree of inventiveness) and possibly redefinition.

Unusual Uses Task : It involves the toy "dog" or the toy "monkey" and requires the subject to redefine the object by giving the cleverest, most interesting, and most unusual uses. The redefinition abilities are considered as required in creative thinking by Guilford and Merrifield (1960). Responses are scored for fluency, flexibility, inventive level, and originality.

(3) Verbal Tasks Using Verbal Stimuli:

Unusual Uses : The unusual uses task using verbal stimuli are direct modifications of Guilford's Brick Uses Test. After preliminary try outs, Torrance (1962) decided to substitute tin for can and books for bricks. Responses are scored for fluency, flexibility and originality.

Impossibilities Task : It is used by Guilford and his associates (1951) as a measure of fluency involving complex restrictions and large potential. In a course in personality development and mental hygiene, Torrance has experimented with a number of modifications of the basic task, making the restrictions more specific. Responses are scored for fluency, flexibility and originality.

Consequences Task : It was chosen by Guilford and his associates (1951) to yield measures both of ideational fluency and penetration. Some examples of improbable situations like "what would happen, if man could become invisible at will?" "What would happen, if a man could live forever on the earth?" be given and the subjects have to think and list their consequences. Responses are scored for fluency, flexibility and originality.

Just Suppose Test: It is an adaptation of the consequences type of test designed to elicit a higher degree of spontaneity and to be more effective with children. As in the consequences task, the subject is confronted with an improbable situation and asked to predict and possible outcomes from the introduction of new or unknown variable. Responses are scored for fluency, flexibility and originality.

Situations Task : These tests were modeled after Guilford's (1951) test designed to assess the ability to see what needs to be done, one of the measures of the factor labelled "sensitivity to problems". Subjects are told that they will be given three common problems and that they be asked to think of as many solutions to these problems as possible. For example, of all schools were abolished, what would you do to try to become educated? Responses are scored for fluency, flexibility and originality.

Common Problems Task : This test is an adaptation of Guilford's (1951) test designed to assess the ability to see defects, needs, and deficiencies and found to be one of the tests of the factor termed "sensitivity to problems". Subjects are instructed that they will be given two common situations and that they will be asked to think of many problems as they can, they might arise in connection with these situations. For examples, doing homework, getting to school on the morning. Responses are scored for fluency, flexibility and originality.

Improvements Tasks: This was adapted from Guilford's (1952) Apparatus Test which was designed to assess ability to see any kind of defects, as aspect of sensitivity to problem. Subjects are asked to think of as many improvements as they can for three common objects. For example a toy dog, ordinary white paper, etc. The general scoring plan for this task is the same as for the situations and common problems.

Mother Hubbard Problem: It was conceived as an adaptation of the situations task for oral administration in the primary grades and also useful in older groups. This test has stimulated a number of ideas concerning factors which inhibit the development of ideas. Responses are scored for fluency and quality.

Cow Jumping Problem: It is comparison task for the Mother Hubbard Problem and has been administered to the same groups, under the same conditions, and scored according to similar procedures. The task is to think of all of the possible things which might have happened when the cow jumped over the moon.

Imaginative Stories: In this task the child is told to write "the most interesting and exciting story" he can think of. Topics are suggested (e.g.: the dog that did not bark) or the child may use his own ideas. The compositions are scored for organisation, sensitivity, originality, psychological insight and richness.

Other Tasks: Several other tasks have been developed for assessing the creative thinking abilities and evaluating creative growth. Those are as follows:

a) Picture Titles: In the picture construction and incomplete figures tasks, subjects will be asked to make up interesting titles for their pictures. Procedures are developed for scoring these for their pictures. Procedures are developed for scoring these for originality and synthesis. It is also planned to have subjects write stories about their pictures.

b) Make-up Problems: Following the design of Getzels and Jackson (1958), simple sets of data are prepared with the instructions to make up as many problems as possible which could be solved with the data supplied. One is a mathematics problem and the other a social studies problem.

c) *Filling-in-gaps:* This task is designed to provide a measure of sensitivity to problems. It consists of a set of the first and last frames of a series of cartoons. The subject's problem is to formulate hypothesis concerning possible intervening events which would follow from the first and results is the last.

d) *Creative Activities Checklists:* Several checklists and inventories of activities, life experiences, and the like have been developed. One is a list of activities which children do on their own in various fields. Another is an inventory of reading interests and habits, and still another is a set of life experience inventories composed of items hypothesized as being related to creative growth. The checklists include activities related to language, art, science, social studies and other fields.

Wallach and Kogan's Contribution

Wallach and Kogan (1965) based their test on the formation of associative elements into combination which are related to creative behaviour. The items are graded from simple to complex. The child answers the questions like a play situation under verbal and non-verbal condition. It mostly measures originality and fluency. A brief note on the tests follows:

1. **Instances Task:** This is the first of three verbal techniques. In this task the child is asked to generate possible instances of a class concept that is specified in verbal times. It is introduced with the general instructions. The child is given as much time as he wishes for each item.

2. **Alternate Uses Task:** This is the second of three verbal techniques. The child is asked to generate possible uses for a verbally specified object.

3. **Similarities Task:** In these test, the child is asked to generate possible similarities between two verbally specified objects.

4. **Pattern Meanings Task:** This is one of the two creativity assessment techniques involving visual rather than verbal stimulus materials.

5. **Line Meanings Task:** In this the child is confronted with one or another kind of line drawings and is asked to generate

meanings or interpretations relevant to the form of the line in question.

For all these tasks, the variables of uniqueness of responses and number of responses are scored.

Identification and measurement of creativity has attracted the attention of Indian investigators, although, in most cases, the measuring tools used were those developed in the United States, particularly those devised by Torrance and Wallach and Kogan.

Several reviews of creativity research have been attempted (Raina, 1969,1971) which consistently show the Torrance's instruments were indeed most popular and translated into various Indian languages. Gakhar and Luthra (1973) examined the test-retest reliability of the Torrance Test of Creative Thinking and the analysis revealed almost consistent high reliability coefficient of correlation for the complete battery.

Basu and Jawa (1973) attempted a factor analytic study of the Torrance Tests of Creative Thinking and the results suggested that Torrance Test of Creative Thinking measure some combination of non-verbal ability and verbal ability. The first factor had appreciable high loadings for figural flexibility, originality and elaboration. This factor was labelled as figural creative ideational ability. The second factor had high loadings for verbal fluency, flexibility, originality and elaboration. This factors was labelled a verbal creative ideational ability. Analyses of these factors like factor 1 revealed that they also involved production of ideas in one form of the other but required verbal ability.

It is, therefore, clear that the verbal and figural tests of creative thinking are not measures of the same creative ability, on the contrary they measure two different abilities. The results suggest that to set a fair and objective picture of creativity as defined by Torrance both the forms—verbal and figural should be used.

The Wallach Kogan instruments were found to be applicable to all age levels. These tests have shown a high degree of internal consistency and are relatively independent of intelligence. Almost all the reported Spearman-Brown reliabilities are varying between 0.80 and 0.93.

Quite a good number of tests of creativity were developed in India during the seventies (Passi, 1972; Paramesh 1972; Mehdi, 1973; Chauhan and Tiwari, 1974; Kaul, 1973; Kaul, 1973; Majumdar, 1973; Kundley, 1977; Ahmed, 1977; Venkata Rami Reddy and Balakrishna Reddy, 1983; and Bakshi, 1986). Most of these tests are based on Guilford's conceptualization of Creative Thinking or on the lines of Torrance's Test model. Many of them measure general creativity but some are developed to measure creativity in specific areas of content.

Passi (1972) developed a battery of creativity tests to measure verbal and non-verbal factors of creativity of the higher secondary school students. The battery consists of six sub-test (both verbal and non-verbal) namely, (i) the Seeing Problems Tests, (ii) the Unusual Uses Test, (iii) the Consequences Test, (iv) the Test of Inquisitiveness, (v) the Square Puzzle Test and (vi) the Blocks Tests of Creativity. Fifteen different scores like fluency, flexibility, originality, persistency etc. can be derived from the test battery.

Parmesh (1972) adapted the Wallach and Kogan tests suitable to Indian culture and found to be valid.

Mehdi (1973) developed a test of creative thinking with verbal and non-verbal components and standardized it on Indian students. In this test creativity tasks pertaining to four factors namely, fluency, flexibility, originality and elaboration were used. This test battery follows the pattern of Torrance's Test of Creative Thinking. It consists of four verbal tests viz., Consequences, Unusual Uses, New Relationships and Product Improvement and Three non-verbal tests viz., Picture Construction, Incomplete Figures, Triangles and Ellipses.

Most of the creativity tests in India are developed for the Doctoral studies. Some of them are published and now are commercially available e.g., Mehdi (1973) and Chauhan and Tiwari (1974).

Kaul (1973) developed a test of creativity for children of 14 to 16 years. The test has items on : sentence completion, uses, creative writing, consequences and problem solving.

Majumdar (1973) developed a test of creativity test battery to measure scientific creativity for the Science Talent Search Scheme of NCERT, New Delhi. Whereas Kundley (1977) developed his creativity test in Marathi to assess literary creativity of the school children.

Ahmed (1977) has reported a study undertaken to develop a battery of creativity tests which could be used as instruments for assessing creativity among children studying in Indian Schools.

Venkata Rami Reddy and Balakrishna Reddy (1983) developed a creativity test battery consisting of 10 sub-tests: (i) Unusual Uses, (ii) Instances, (iii) Similarities, (iv) Common Problems, (v) Impossibilities (vi) Consequences, (vii) Product Improvement (viii) Pattern meanings, (ix) Line meanings, and (x) Circles Test. These tests were in line with those constructed by Getzels and Jackson (1962), Torrance (1963) and Wallach and Kogan (1965). The first seven sub-tests were verbal while the remaining were non-verbal. The split-half reliability of the different sub-tests scored for fluency, flexibility and originality which ranged between 0.75 and 0.99; as there was only one item in the "impossibilities test", the split-half reliability could not be established. The test battery was administered to the sample of students in small groups in a game like manner (Wallach and Kogan, 1965), without any time limit.

Bakshi (1986) constructed a test batter to identify creative behaviour in 4 and 5 year olds. The test battery contains four measures of fluency, flexibility, elaboration and originality, and two measures of fantasy, predisposition. Then subjected to validation and internal consistency testing procedures. It predicts original problem solving as assessed buy Moran, et al's (1983) multidimensional test battery and performance on the circles task, a subject common to Torrance's (1968) measures of figural creativity and the new test battery. Teacher's ratings were found to be an inadequate external criterion. Computations of internal consistency suggested that the maths work page should not be retained in the test battery.

Contributions to the Measurement of Field Dependence/Independence Cognitive Style

Individuals respond to different situations based on their particular cognitive style. A variety of tests have been used to measure the characteristics of cognitive style. The important and commonly used measures of field dependence/independence are Embedded Figures Test (EFT) and Rod-and-Frame Test (RET). These tests were developed by Witkin, et al (1954).

In Embedded Figures Test, the subject is asked to locate a simple figure embedded in a complex geometric form. His score is the mean time taken to locate the simple figures for 24 test items. Those who find the simple form quickly are labelled field independents and those

who have difficult are labelled field dependents.

Different forms of Embedded Figures Test are (1) children's Embedded Figures Test (CEFT), (2) Group Embedded Figures Test (GEFT) and (3) Preschool Embedded Figures Test (PEFT). A brief account of these tests is as follows:

(1) The children's Embedded Figures Test developed by Goodenough and Eagle (1963), is a modified version of the EFT designed for use with children. As in the EFT, the subject from which the simple figures may be removed. The score is the number of simple figures correctly identified. It has been standardized for children 5 to 9 years of age. The reliability of the CEFT ranges from 0. 72 to 0.90 (Saracho, 1980, 1983, 1984).

(2) The 24-items Group Embedded Figures Test was developed by Witkin, et al (1972). The subjects task is to find the simple form in the complex figures. This test has eight simple geometric forms that are embedded within more complex stimulus patterns. The scores range from 0 to 18 correct, with higher scores suggesting more field independent functioning. It is an accuracy based measure rather than a time-based measure.

(3) The pre School Embedded Figures Test is also a form of the EFT which measures field dependence/independence. It was developed by Coates (1972) by adapting the Children's Embedded Figures Test for children 3 to 5 years of age by eliminating the colour in the figures and decreasing the number of distracting simple forms in a complex figure.

In Standard Rod-and-Farme Test, the subject is seated in a light proof frame and rod tilted, he is asked to adjust the rod to the objective upright. The RFT is divided into three series: where the subject's chair is tilted opposite to the tilt of the frame; where the subject's chair is tilted to the same side as the frame; where the subject is seated erect. The score for each series is the mean number of degrees of deviation of the rod from the upright when the subject sees it in straight. Four counter balanced trials of the dark room version (frame sides subtend 28° of visual angle) are given with subject's viewing the frame tilted 22.5° clockwise and counter clockwise from an upright body position (mean on this test = + 6.7°).

Different forms of Rod-and-Frame Test are mentioned as follows:

1. Body-tilted RET was developed by Witkin, et al (1954). The body tilted to the side by 20° clock-wise or counter clock-wise. Since the vertical task cannot be translated into an egocentric task when the body is tilted, this variable is included to further explore the role of strategy choice eliminating the option of aligning the rod with the head (mean = + 9.1).

2. Tilting Room - Tilting Chair Test was developed by Witkin, et al (1954). The subject is seated in a chair within a specially constructed room. The room and Chair can be tilted independently to the right or left. At the beginning of each of the 14 trials, the room and chair are tilted. For the first 8 trials, called the Room Adjustment Test (RAT), the subject is asked to adjust the tilted room to the upright, while the chair remains tilted. The remaining trials, called the Body Adjustment Test (BAT), involve adjustment of the chair (and thus as subject's body) to the upright while the room remains tilted. Both RAT and BAT are divided into two series. Series I of each test include trials where room and chair are initially tilted to opposite sides and series II where they are tilted to the same side. For each series of each test the subject's score is the mean deviation in degrees, of his estimates from the true upright.

3. Supine RET was developed by Rock (1975), and Timpleton (1973). Subjects are asked to align the rod egocentrically while viewing an overhead RET from the supine body position. Since the gravitational direction is irrelevant to the definition of to tilt in a horizontal plane, individual difference vertical.

4. Small lit-room RFT: A display of small visual angle (frame sides subtending 9° of visual angle) tilted by 15° was shown in a lit room. Visual effects on vestibular responses should be slight to non-existent, but systematic errors can be produced under conditions of this sort (Gosel and Newton, 1975; Coren and Hoy, 1986).

5. Zollner version was developed by Oyarna (1975). The display consists of eight series of slides. The slides in each series show two long lines at varying orientation, on which is crossed by shorter lines at an angle of 22.5°. The subject's task is to select from each series the one side in which the long lines look most nearly parallel. It is dropped after the first 97 subjects.

6. **Egocentric RET was developed by Sigman, et al (1979). Instructions to align the rod with the longitudinal axis of the body are substituted for the standard instructions to align the rod with the gravitational vertical. It is dropped after the first 97 subjects.**
7. **Small-dark-room RFT: This test is added after the first 97 subjects. It is identical to the small lit room RFT except that the rod and frame are the only visible stimuli. The dark room version is developed to eliminate vertical and horizontal lines in the lit room that may dilute or inhibit the contrast effect.**
8. **Portable Rod-and-Frame Test was devised by Nickel (1971). This test is a portable version of the test used by Witkin and his colleagues (1962), to define the cognitive style and field-articulation. Although the task is perceptual (to overcome the distorting effect of the tilted frame in order to align a luminous rod vertically, with no other visual cues available), inferences about a general cognitive style have been made because of the many relationships found with personality and ability variables.**

Among all Rod-and-Frame Tests, Tilting-Room Tilting-Chair Test, Portable Rod-and-Frame Test are mostly used measures.

The different forms of the Embedded Figures Test and the Rod-and-Frame Test can be used with children but both are individually administered, time consuming, and expensive. Goodenough-Harris Drawing Test and the Articulation of the Body Concept Scale eliminate these difficulties.

The Goodenough-Harris Drawing Test (Harris, 1963) is designed to measure conceptual thinking. Children draw pictures of a male and a female which are scored for details present. The mean of scores on both the male and female drawings is used to obtain a higher reliability.

Witkin, et al (1974) developed an Articulation of the Body Concept Scale to assess field dependence/independence. It is administered to children in a group by asking them to draw a picture of a male on a paper and picture of a female on another paper. A minium of two judges must independently rate the set of drawings on a five-point scale based on (a) the form level of drawings. (b) the degree to which the identity and sex are differentiated in the drawing, and (c) the level of detailing in the drawing.

Contributions to the Measurement of Reflection/impulsivity Cognitive Style

The instrument most often used to measure reflection/impulsivity is the Matching Familiar Figures Test (MFFT). It was developed by Kogan, et al (1954). Different forms of the MFFT are available for pre-schoolars, school age children, and adults. The MFFT is a match-to-standard test consisting of 12 test items and two sample items. Each item consists of a standard drawing and six alternative drawings which are very similar to the standard. The subject is shown the standard and the alternatives simultaneously and is instructed to one of the alternatives that exactly matches the standard. When the subject's first response is incorrect, he is told to combine choosing alternatives until he selects the correct one. The elapsed time between the presentation of the item and the completion of the subject's first response is recorded and summed across all 12 test items. The total number of errors is also tallied. The latency and error scores, on the MFFT are both used as measures of the subject's cognitive tempo.

Block, et al (1974) and Ault, et al (1975) reported an internal consistency, reliability coefficient for MFFT responses times of 0.89 but lower reliabilities of 0.62 and 0.58 respectively, for errors. The unpublished data of several researchers collected by Ault, et al (1975). Yielded typical internal consistency reliabilities for MFFT errors is the 0.50.

Among pre-school children, MFFT errors are moderately stable overtime, whereas response time is not stable. By contrast, among school age children, response time is moderately stable over time but errors are not.

Rather low reliability of MFFT errors in school age children as measured by short-term test-retest reliability, internal consistency reliability, or stability over longer periods of time-results in several problems (Ault, et al., 1975). One of these problems is mis-classification of subjects among the four conceptual tempo groups (reflective, impulsive, fast-accurate and slow-inaccurate.

Although such problems with the MFFT exist, a different strategy might be to refine the test in such a way as to increase it's reliability.

Similar Matching Familiar Figures Tests- Those containing fewer variants—have recently been developed for use with younger children (Banta, 1970; Lewis, Rausch and Goldberg, 1968 and Wright, 1971). Of these, the Kansas Reflection/impulsivity scale for pre schoolers (KRISP) (Wright, 1971, 1973) has been developed and studied most systematically. It is administered individually to each subject. These are two comparable forms of KRISP each consisting of 5 practice items followed by 10 test items. Basically the child is simply asked to find that number of the lower array which exactly matches the standard above. The child is timed in seconds till the first response whether correct or wrong. If he makes at the first response, he is given two more trials. Norms, reliability data, and age and sex differences for this instrument, along with a preliminary investigation of scanning strategies of impulsive and reflective, were reported by McClusky and Wright (1973). The smaller negative correlation between response time and errors (about-0.11) and the stability of conceptual tampo over 1 year in young boys suggest that the either the KRISP is not a measure of reflection/impulsivity.

Yando and Kagan (1970) constructed 10 different Matching Familiar Figures Tests and administered to 7- year-olds, one test each week for 10 weeks. Inspite of differences in task complexity, which were accompanied by increases in response time and errors, most children retained their relative rank on both response time and errors. The median correlation over 10 weeks was 0.73 for response time and 0.68 for errors, Similarly, Ward (1968) administered two different matching tests to kindergarten children—one with three response alternative and one with five alternatives- made up of geometrical or meaningful figures. Response times on the two tests inter-correlated 0.64 for males and 0.57 for females.

Two other tests used to explore the generality of reflection/ impulsivity are the Design Recall Test (DRT) and the Haptic Visual Matching Test (HVMT) (Kagan, et al., 1964) In the DRT, the standard and alternatives are geometrical forms rather than familiar objects, and the subject must choose the correct alternative from his memory of the standard, which is viewed first and then removed. The standard in the HVMT is either a three-dimensional geometrical form or a familiar object that the subject feels but does not see; the correct alternative is also chosen from memory. Response times to the MFFT, DRT, and HVMT are moderately inter-correlated, raging from 0.33 to 0.52 (Kagan, 1965 and Kagan et al., 1966).

Summing up, the reflection/impulsivity construct remains robust over changes in the MFFT, it also extends to tests containing different requirements and content.

STUDIES ON INTER-RELATION BETWEEN CREATIVITY AND COGNITIVE STYLES

Studies on Inter-Relation between Creativity and Field Dependence/ Independence Cognitive Style

Western Studies

Some of the researchers studies about the interrelation between creativity and field dependence/independence cognitive style. Getzels and Jackson's (1962) study revealed that high creative and high intelligence groups correspond to Witkin's independent and dependent cognitive style respectively. Indeed, many of the qualities of the creative divergent thinker, and of the child-rearing conditions which encourage creativity, are similar to those attributed to the field independence.

A number of study by Bloomberg, Spotts and Mackler (1967) have appeared supporting the theoretical relationship of the field independent cognitive style to creative test performance. It was found that, while all subjects who score high on field independence are not necessarily creative, those scoring high on various measures of creativity tend to score significantly higher in field independence.

Spotts and Mackler (1967) gave two verbal and two non-verbal creativity tests and two versions of Embedded Figures Test (for field independent/dependent cognitive style) to 114 male students, and obtained small but fairly consistent correlations with the various Torrance creativity scores.

McWhinnie's (1967) study obtained scarcely any significant correlation among 6th graders between Embedded Figures Test (to measure field independent/dependent cognitive style) and several art and creativity tests.

Eagles, Goldberger and Beritman (1969); Fitzgibbons and Goldberger (1971) found that field dependent individuals attend more to verbal information with social connotations.

Goldberger and Bendich (1972) found that there is a positive correlation between field dependence and the generation of social words during an unstructured free association task.

Kaufman (1975) found significant relationship between Embedded Figures Test measured field independence/dependence cognitive style and Torrance Test of Creativity composite score.

Goodenough (1976) found that there is a tendency of field dependent subjects to use passive or spectator approaches in problem-solving situations.

Witkin, Moore, Goodenough and Cox (1977) found that field independent persons find it easier to solve tasks involving functional fixity than do field dependent persons.

Noppe (1977) studied the relationship between Remote Association Test (for creativity) and Embedded Figures Test (for field independent/dependent cognitive style). It was found that field independent subjects were more creative than field dependent subjects.

Morris and Bergum (1978) examined the potential relation ship between career choice as a predictor of creativity and individual scores on a measure of field dependence and field independence. Two groups of undergraduates, 13 Architectural and 25 Business students at Texas A & M University, took the short form of the Witkin Group Embedded Figures Test (According to Bergum's (1977) study, students in architecture tend to see themselves as being more creative than do students in business). Results indicate that a significant difference between two groups with the architectural students showing more field independence. Such results suggest that students choosing more creative careers tend to be more field independent.

Linn (1978) found that field dependence/independence is associated with logical reasoning.

Frank and Noble (1985) study investigated the hypothesis that field independent individuals are more efficient in their use of cognitive restructuring skills than are field dependent individuals. Thirty two field independent and thirty two field dependent female under-graduates were required to solve a series of anagrams under either an easy or difficult anagram condition. Each individual received five anagrams constructed from "social" words and five anagrams constructed from "non-social" words. The results of the analysis of anagram performance supported the belief that field independent individuals find it easier than field dependent individuals to provide a disorganized field with organization. Field independents solved the anagrams significantly quicker than did field dependent students.

Smilansky and Halberstadt (1986) found field independence cognitive style exhibited in creative problem solving.

Harritte (1987) conducted a study to determine the strength of the relationships between field independence/dependence, visualization, and problem solving in adolescent males and females. Hundred, 8th graders were administered the Group Embedded Figures Test (GEFT), Pursue Perceptual Screening Test (PPST) and Cognitive Abilities Test and Verbal Problems test to measure field independence/ dependence, visualization and problem solving ability respectively. Subjects who were field independent and highly visual and field dependent with low visualization were identified. Then, the relationship between these subjects cognitive style and problem solving was examined. Statistical analysis revealed that problem solving was positively related to cognitive style and visualization. Field-independent subjects with high visualization scored higher than field dependent subjects with low visualization on both problem-solving measures. Males were fund to be more field independent than females. Males scored higher than females on the embedded figures task and the relationship between part one of the PPST and the GEFT were highly correlated for females.

Indian Studies

Rastogi (1978) investigated the difference in intellectual level and creativity of 30 male and 30 female field independent or field dependent Indian adults. Creativity but not intelligence was associated with cognitive style: sex and the interaction between sex and cognitive style did not significantly affect creativity or intelligence levels.

Bal (1988) studied the relationship between creativity, cognitive styles and academic achievement. The sample of 150 high, middle, low academic achievers (age range of 18-21 years) from various colleges of Delhi were selected. Embedded Figures Test was used to measure cognitive style (field independence/dependence), Torrance Test of Creative Thinking (TTCT) verbal Form A and Remote Association Test (RAT) were administered to measure creativity. The analysis of variance of the creativity scores on various measures revealed that both field independent cognitive style and academic achievement are related to fluency, flexibility and originality scores of TTCT as well as creativity measured by RAT. It was also observed that field independent cognitive style and academic achievement significantly interact with RAT creativity and not with TTCT creativity.

Studies on Inter-Relation between Creativity and Reflection/ impulsivity Cognitive Style

Western studies

Kagan, Person and Welch (1966) found that reflective children performed better than impulsive children on tasks of reasoning.

Kagan (1966) found that reflective revealed better, short-term auditory memory on a serial learning task than did impulsive.

Ward (1968) found that the cognitive style reflection/impulsivity was unrelated to creativity, although hypothesized antecedents of this dimension are identical to those which have been proposed for various creativity subgroups.

Shipe (1971) and Weintraub (1973) found reflectives solved proteus maze more successfully than impulsive.

Kagan and Kogan (1970) and Block, et al's (1974) study indicated that impulsive children, as compared to reflective children demonstrate poor academic achievement and poor performance on a variety of problem-solving tasks.

Fuque, Bartsch, and Phye (1975) investigated the relationship between cognitive tempo and creativity in preschool age children. The subjects were 70 enrolled in a large urban nursery school located in Central Iowa. A modified version of the Kagan's Matching Familiar Figures Test were used to measure creativity and reflection/impulsivity cognitive style respectively. A significant effect for cognitive tempo was found showing reflective subjects scoring higher than impulsive subjects on each measure of creativity.

Haskins ,and McKinney (1976) studied the relative effects of response tempo and accuracy on problem solving. To examine the relationship between response accuracy and tempo, as measured by the Matching Familiar Figures Test (MFFT) and criterion measures, 233 7, 9 and 11 year-old children were given the MFFT, 2 problem-solving tasks and test of academic achievement, univarate correlations between the MFFT variables and the problems-solving and academic achievement variables revealed a number of significant correlations involving MFFT errors but relatively few significant correlations involving MFFT latency. Multiple regression demonstrated that MFFT variable did not add substantially to the univariate correlations.

Klein, Blockovich, Buchalter and Huyghe (1976) studied the relationship between reflectio~/impulsivity and problem solving. Performance of 88 children cat rized as reflective or impulsive was compared on convergent and divergent problem solving tasks. The Matching Familiar Figures Test was administered along with the tests for determining the correct order or a word sequence, and for listing unusual uses for familiar objects. Reflective children (n = 33) made significantly fewer errors on the convergent problem solving task than impulsive children (n = 33) but th ere was no effect of cognitive style on the divergent problem solving task.

Adejumo's (1979) purpose of the study was to find the degree and nature of relationship between the tempo of response and accuracy on problem-solving tasks as measured by modified matching familiar figures and performance on visual perceptual tasks. Two hundred male subjects draw from age group of 7 and 9 years olds (n = 100 each) in classes 2 and 4 respectively, were classified into four groups (impulsive, reflective, fast-accurate, slow-inaccurate) based on performance on modified Matching Familiar Figures Test. Subjects were also tested on object-comparison and visual recognition tasks performance on modified matching familiar figures correlate significantly with performance on visual perceptual task (r = 0.58 and 0.63 for 7 and 9 year olds, respectively). Seven year old subjects in the reflective and fast-accurate groups were superior in performance on the visual perceptual tasks.

Sigg and Gargiulo (1980) studied the creativity and cognitive style in 42 learning disabled and 44 non-disabled students. They were administered the Matching Familiar Figures Test and the Torrance Test of Creative Thinking. A chi-square analysis suggested a significant difference between the cognitive styles of the two groups of children. Multivariable analysis of variance indicate no significant differences in creativity between learning disabled and non-disabled students or between reflective and impulsive individuals. Correlational analysis suggested that errors and latencies on the Matching Familiar Figures

Test were not significantly related to the creative abilities of either learning disabled or non-disabled children.

INFLUENCE OF DEMOGRAPHIC FACTORS ON CREATIVITY AND COGNITIVE STYLES

Studies on Ethnicity and Creativity

Western Studies

Social class and race also influence divergent thinking (creativity) but the results are complex. In his samples of black and white pre school children from varying socio economic levels, Saveca (1965) found that the high socio economic groups scored significantly higher than the low ones on total divergent thinking. There was also a significant interaction between race and IQ; that is, high IQ black children scored higher than low IQ black children but the reverse was true of white children. Scores for verbal and non-verbal aspects of divergent thinking appear to differentiate social classes and black and white children.

Smith (1965) found that among fifth-grade white children in Pittsburgh, the middle-class performed significantly better on verbal tasks, but the lower-class excelled on non-verbal items.

In a group of Texas lower-class white and black children 5 to 9 years of age, who were individually given Torrance's Unusual Uses Test and the Wechsler intelligence Scale for Children (WISC), Iscoe and Pierce-Jones (1965), found that black children generally obtained higher divergent thinking scores, primarily in terms of ideational fluency, but the white children got significantly higher IQ scores on the WISC. In both races, there were significant correlations between creativity and intelligence (0.25 for blacks, 0.28 for whites).

Douing (1970) studied a group of 7th grade Australian children from 10 Metropolitan schools. They were given tests of divergent thinking, intelligence and academic achievement. A highly significant relationship was found for mean creativity scores for each school and the socio economic level of the district.

Bhan (1970) observed that creativity index did not significantly differentiate different social class subjects.

Hurlock (1981) stated that children from higher socio-economic groups tend to be more creative than those of the lower socio economic groups tend to be more creative than those of the lower socio economic status a there are more opportunities for giving the knowledge and experience necessary for creativity. The former for the most part are brought up under democratic child training methods while the latter for more likely to experience authoritarian training. Democratic control fosters creativity by giving children more opportunities to express their individuality and pursue interests and activities of their own choice.

Doyle (1970) hypothesized that Negroes would exhibit creative talents superior to that of their Cancasian classroom peers and observed that the hypothesis was not statistically supported, though there was a tendency towards Negroes superiority on the creativity measures. But, Ridhmond (1971) observed that the cancasian students were significantly higher (0.05 level) on verbal and non-verbal intelligence, verbal fluency, verbal flexibility, figural flexibility and figural originality. No difference between Negro and White children in respect to their creativity scores were found in the studies conducted by Halpin, Halpin and Torrance (1973).

Indian Studies

Raina's (1968) study designed to compare significant difference between high and low creative groups on selected measures of cognition, personality and socio economic status. Minnesota Tests of Creative Thinking was administered to a total population of 500 students of three educational zones of Rajasthan, 100 high and 100 low score were delineated. Only 90 in the former group (high creative) and 85 in the latter (low creative) were available for the final analysis. The results revealed the significant differences between the IQs of the two groups, differences being in favour of high creative. Significant differences were noted in the socio economic status of the high creative on all three dimensions of the socio economic status scale used.

Sowjanya (1974) and Ahmed (1980) found that creatives came from higher socio economic strata.

Badarinath and Satyanarayana (1970) Chandha and Sen (1981) and Venkata Rami Reddy and Tulsi Devi (1981) reported that there was no significant difference in the creativity of students belonging to high, middle and low socio economic groups.

Kundu and Mallick (1987) studied the factors affecting creativity and found that socio economic status is an important factor in fostering creativity. The influence upon the person's creativity ability may be both positive and negative. From the very nature of the inner conditions of an individual, it is evident that creativity cannot be forced but may be stimulated to emerge and there may be an optimum level under the favourable environmental conditions.

Ahmed and Joshi (1978) studied the impact of socio-cultural disadvantage on Mehdi's Non-Verbal Creative Thinking in 120 students from advantaged and disadvantaged schools, advantaged and disadvantaged homes and 7th, 9th and 11th grade. Results revealed that home and school differences were important only at the 7th grade level, whereas the combined effects of the two environments were significant through 11th grade. At higher grade level, irrespective of the type of schools, there occurred a more rapid increase in creativity scores of disadvantaged subjects as compared to their advantaged counterparts.

Ahmed (1980) studied the effect of socio cultural disadvantage on creative thinking, verbal and non-verbal creativity tests were administered to 150, 8th, 9th and 10th graders in 5 Indian schools that were on a continuum from extremely advantaged to extremely disadvantaged. Subjects were classified as being from advantaged and disadvantaged home backgrounds; significant main effects of grade, school and home background were found on the creative thinking tests, and all interactions were significant except for the grade and school interaction.

Cognitive-affective abilities and social backgrounds of tribal and non-tribal primary school dropouts were studied by Yadav and Dash (1980). In a 2 × 2 × 2 factorial design, drop-out and regular children (N = 80) belonging to tribal and non-tribal population residing in rural areas and reading in 3rd and 5th graders were tested. Questionnaires and tests were the tools used. Results revealed that the drop-out had lower intelligence scores, were found to be less creative had limited vocabulary and poor linguistic ability, showed lower achievement motivational levels, were found to be impulsive and lacking flexibility. Their families were found to be less effective in satisfying their needs.

Krishna Kumari, Lalitha and Parmaji (1986) conducted a study in Warangal, Andhra Pradesh to compare the creativity of tribal (Lambada, Koya and Yerukala) children with that of the non-tribal children. The sample was 50 boys and 50 girls of class VIII. Mehdi's Test of Creative Thinking was used to measure verbal and non-verbal components of creativity. Results revealed that the tribal children were deficient in regard to the level of verbal creative thinking (originality fluency, flexibility and elaboration). The performance of tribal children in non-verbal creativity (originality and elaboration) test were superior to the non-tribal children.

Golwalder (1986) studied the scientific attitude, creativity and achievement of tribal students of Rajasthan. The sample consisted of 270 tribal and 270 non-tribal students of IX and X classes offering science as optional subjects and living in tribal areas. Mehdi's Verbal and Non-verbal Test of Creative Thinking was used for measuring creativity. This test consists of fluency, flexibility, originality and elaboration components. Results reported that in verbal creativity, the non-tribals excelled the tribals in all components except flexibility and in non-verbal creativity the performance on non-tribals was better in all components without any exception.

The effect of parent's educational level and economic status on creativity of the Adivasi female students was studied by Asifa (1986). It was found that parent's economic condition had a significant effect upon the creativity. The higher creative group found in the upper economic group and the lower creative group in the lower economic group. Parent's education had no effect upon the creativity scores.

Sharma (1972) conducted a study to find out the rural-urban differences in creative thinking. Two tests of creativity namely Srujanatmakta Pariksha and Varna Viparyas Pariksha were administered to X class male students from urban and rural areas. The results showed there was no significant difference in creativity between rural and urban students.

Sharma (1974), in a study of creativity as a function of intelligence, Fine Art Interest and Culture, employing 2 × 2 × 2 factorial design, found creativity to be affected by all the three factors and their interactions, except for the interaction of Fine Art Interest and Culture. He observed that high level of intelligence was necessary for creative thinking. Importance of rural culture was shown by the fact that goals of expressive group (rural) were easily approachable and clear, whereas the oppressive group (urban) had to play individual roles to achieve their life goals.

Cross Cultural Studies

Cross cultural comparisons are valuable since they facilitate an understanding of the impact and interaction of different environmental influence on behaviour.

Torrance (1968) made a comparative study of the performance of various cultural groups on tests of creative thinking. It was found that children from highly developed cultures scored better on elaboration than children from the less developed cultures such as the U.S. Negro Group, Western Samoa and India. The children in India performed disproportionately better on verbal than on figural tests. Indian boys scored higher than girls in verbal tests but not on figural ones.

Trowbridge (1968) studied children from India, Afghanistan, Iraq and Lebanon. They were asked to describe two of their novel ideas including the conditions under which they occurred, with whom he had shared it, the reaction of others to it. Sex and cultural differences were noted. Ideas described any girls were generally in the area of arts and crafts and communication, whereas boys dealt primarily with mechanical arts and agriculture; Indian children, in contrast to those from the Middle East had more ideas when relaxed, shared their ideas less often, had fewer intellectual type ideas and evidenced less inner satisfaction.

A cross cultural research was undertaken by Singh (1970) to compare American and Indian subject's creative abilities. Matfessal Individual Tests of Creativity were used to measure creativity. Data was gathered from Tempa and Banaras. Results revealed that disadvantaged children, regardless of culture, did not score low on the verbal part of the creativity test, and with an increase in socio economic status, abilities, such as flexibility and originality excelled at the cost of redefinition, fluency, sensitivity to problems elaboration.

Ogletree and Ujlaki (1973) in a cross cultural study of English, Scottish and German subjects observed that creativity scores were function of socio economic background. They further observed that in all countries subjects from upper class families obtained significant higher creative scores (verbal and non-verbal) than subjects from middle and lower class families.

Studies on Ethnicity and Field Dependence/Independence Cognitive Style

Many writers have attributed the different ways of perceiving things by different individuals to such factors as the environment in which a person grows up, the gender of the individual and the child rearing practices operative in the cultures. A number of studies on cognitive style have been carried out in relation to social values, social consensus, child rearing practices, ecology and acculturation.

Western Studies

Berry (1966) found that the Eskimos and Arunta, two non-industrialized societies to be relatively field-independent. These groups, although non-industrialized and presumably "primitive" share with industrialized societies the small nuclear family, permissive child rearing practices and high levels of mobility. Thus there are apparently several factor other than social traditionalism which determine cognitive sty e in various and economic environments.

Okonji (1969) found a significant difference on Rod-and-Frame Test between Nigerian adolescents of rural and urban background undergraduates giving more differentiated performance.

Smith (1971) studied acculturation and field dependence among the Xhosa. Rod-and-Frame Test was administered to 3 xhosa groups (n=30) of varying levels of acculturation under graduates, urban dwellers, and rural reserve dwellers and to 30 white undergraduates. Results supported earlier research and suggested that development of the analytic cognitive style of the field independent personality is facilitated by democratic socialization practices and well developed habits of perceptual analysis common among acculturated groups.

Marjoribanks (1978) studied the ehnicity, family environment and cognitive performance. The sample consisted of 850, 11 years old girls and boys from Australian ethnic groups. They have seen the relations, between scores on a new family environment interview schedule and the intelligence, mathematics, word knowledge and word comprehension. Results indicated that after accounting for joint effects and the unique influence of the environment, ethnicity generally continued to make small, unique contributions to he variation in cognitive scores.

The effect of rural and urban upbringing on cognitive styles was studied by Tharakan (1987). Group Embedded Figures Test was administered to eighty rural and urban Birom Nigerian under- graduates (the mean age 18; 35 years). Results showed that (a) the subjects who resided in urban environment were more field independent than those in rural environments; (b) urban males were more field independent than the urban females; (c) There were no sex differences in field dependence/independence between the rural male and female Biroms; (d) a marked difference existed in the individuals level of field independence was positively related to the levels of economic development and modernization influences.

Indian Studies

Dash, and Dash (1980) studied perceptual motor and intellectual abilities of tribal and non-tribal pre school children. The sample was of 48 tribal and 48 non-tribal children in the age range of 4-6 years. Three non-verbal tests of intelligence (Raven's Coloured Progressive Matrices, Goodenough-Harris Draw-A Man Test, Columbia Mental Maturity Scale) and Perceptual-Motor Tests (Embedded Figures Test, Figures Matching Test, Grapto-Motor Test and Visual-Motor Integration Test) were administered. The results revealed significant linear trends over age in all test scores for the two groups. However, the development was slower for tribal children. In all the tests the mean scores of the tribal different significantly from those of the non-tribal children.

Research was designed by Mohapatra (1980) for the comparative assessment of the cognitive abilities of the unschooled children (11-12 years) among two primitive tribes (Bonda and Dongria Kandh) of Orissa. The tests administered were (1) Raven's Progressive Matrices Test to measure level of intelligence; (2) to measure cognitive style or linguistic ability, Stroop's Colour-Word Test; (3) basic learning ability by Digit Span Test; (4) Pictorial Concept Formation Test and Figure Copying Test to measure pictorial conception and figure reproduction; and (5) Finger Dexterity Test to measure level of non-verbal aspiration and achievement. Results showed that on the level of intelligence, basic learning ability, pictorial conception and figure copying and on the level of non-verbal aspiration and achievement the Bondas scored higher than the Dongria. On cognitive style the scores for both the groups were on par with each other.

Cross Cultural Studies

Wober (1967) proposed that in African culture, the authority spheres are relatively more important than the visual sphere which is predominant in European and American culture. He demonstrated that

Nigerian subjects when tested with Rod-and-Frame Test with a tilting chair were better able to overcome the effects of tilted chair when adjusting the rod to the vertical position than the American control group.

A comparative study of cognitive styles in 3 ethnic groups was studied by Ghuman (1980). He assessed the test performance of 3 groups; 50 English, 50 West Indians and 50 Asians, whose cultures differ in socialization practices. Subjects were secondary school students (age 12 years 10 months to 13 years 10 months). The Group Embedded Figures Test and Spatial and Mathematics Tests were given to assess performance. Results revealed that the performance of the Asiatic and West Indian subject were significantly inferior to that of the English on the GEFT. Asiatics were significantly superior to the West Indian and English groups on the Mathematics Test . No significant differences appeared between groups on the Spatial Tests, and no sex differences were found.

Saracho's (1983) studies report that field independence is associated with cultural differences.

Shade (1986) examined the possibility of a unique culturally induced Afro-American cognitive style. One hundred and seventy eight 9th grade students stratified by race, sex and achievement level were administered 3 cognitive style tasks (i.e., an Object Sorting Task, the Group Embedded Figures Test, Myers - Briggs Type Indicator). Results revealed a significant difference between Afro-and Euro-American subjects in their perceptual orientation to the environment. Findings suggest that the Blacks were more spontaneous, flexible and open-minded and less-structured in their perceptions of people, events and ideas, while the Euro-Americans appeared to be self-regulated, judgmental and less open-minded. It is suggested that this difference may influence the performance patterns reported on non-verbal measures.

Studies on Ethnicity and Reflection/impulsivity Cognitive Style

Western Studies

Smith and Ribordy (1980) assessed 72 kindergarten males from Chicago, Illionois for reflection/impulsivity with the Matching Familiar Figures Test. Cognitive style on this test was examined in relation to intelligence, socio-economic status, race, father's absence and teacher's ratings of impulsivity. Significant findings included boys whose fathers were absent from the home made more errors on the test than boys whose fathers were prasent in the home. Teachers rated more intelligent boys are more impulsive and these teacher's ratings were positively correlated with errors but not latencies. No significant differences in cognitive style were found for race or socio economic groups.

Cross Cultural Studies

Although cognitive tempo has been studied from a variety of prespectives there is no large-sclae research comparing differences in cognitive tempo (Reflection/impulsivity) among different cultural groups.

Data on the Matching Familiar Figures Test for over 5,000 American, Japanese and Israeli children were used to examine cross-cultural differences in cognitive tempo by Salkind, Kojima and Zelnikes (1978). Factorial analyses of variance revealed significant main effects for age, sex, and nationality as well as age x nationality interactions for both errors and latency. Younger Japanese children made fewer errors than their American or Israeli counterparts and continued to do so until 8 years of age, when their level of accuracy approached that of 10-12 year old American and Israeli children. The age x nationality interaction for latency revealed peak performance for Japanese children at 8 years of age, while the latency for American and Israeli children continued to increase up until about 10, eventually becoming slower than their Japanese counterparts. All three cultual groups tend to be characterized by highly similar developmental trends for both errors and latency, as well as synchrony within each group between peak latency and asymptotic error scores. There also appears to be a developmental shift present, where these patterns are evedenced in Japanese children 2 years earlier than in American and Israeli children.

Cultural differences in cognitive style development were studied by smith and caplan (1988). Children in several cultures seem to develop a similar cognitive style on Matching Familiar then more fast accurate. However, there are two impressions that qualify these account. First, the early MFFT development of Japanese children seems distinctive in that they become far more accurate in the MFFT, with small increase in latency. Second in several cultures, error decreases may dominate latency increases in early development, implying this to MFFT measures cognitive competence as well as cognitive style.

Evaluating either impression requires some way of qualifying speed and accuracy in the MFFT, so that they can be directly compared across age and culture groups. They illustrate such an analysis with the MFFT records of 100 Chinese-American children, age 6-10 and the recognize existing data to compare MFFT performance across four cultures. In all four cultures, error rates decrease more than latency increases. However Japanese children's unique development on the MFFT is supported.

Studies on Age and Creativity

In recent years many research workers have made observations regarding the growth of creative abilities along with age.

Western Studies

Piers, et al(1960) reported that creativity test scores tend to increase with chronological age, a finding not substantiated by Torrance (1964) who reported, on the basis of Minnesota Tests of Creative Ability, that creative abilities decline between sixth and seventh grades, then rise steadily until near the end of high school, after which they level off and decline slightly.

Olshin (1965) reported significant positive relationship between age and verbal creativity test scores (order subjects and higher means than younger subjects) but the relationship did not hold for non-verbal tests.

Trowbridge and Charles (1966) found that technical competence increases gradually and steadily with age, and creativity remains relatively constant from 3 to 15 years with a sharp rise from 15 to 18 years.

Indian Studies

Passi (1972) observed significant development trends of creativity scores along grades from nine through eleventh. Similar results were obtained by Venkata Rami Reddy and Balakrishna Reddy (1984).

Paramesh (1970) and Sowjanya (1974) found that there was no significant effect of age on creativity.

Badarinath and Satyanarayana (1979) reported that creativity increased up to the age of 13 years.

A significant development in the verbal and non-verbal creativity from classes VII to XI was reported by Ahmed (1980).

Joshi (1974), Gakhar (1975) and Dharmangadan (1981) found that creativity increased upto the age of 15 years.

Venkata Rami Reddy and Balakrishna Reddy (1984) observed that creativity increased from class VIII to X.

Raina (1970) and Venkata Rami Reddy and Saleema (1988) observed that creativity and age were positively and significantly related to each other.

Studies on Sex Differences and Creativity

The different creative potentials have been marked among persons due to individual differences. These differences have been considered due to age factor, aptitude and interest of the individual sex differences etc.

Research findings about sex differences on creativity are varied and their results are not conclusive. There are three contradictory trends observable in these findings.

1. Boys are superior to girls in creative thinking.
2. Girls are superior to boys in creative thinking, and
3. There is no sex difference in creativity ability.

1. Studies Reporting Boys are Highly Creative:

Western Studies

Kelly (1965) and Middents (1968) observed males scoring higher than females on non-verbal creativity measures in their samples of school and college students.

Starus and Straus (1968) reported that boys performed better than girls on measures of creativity in both Indian and American Culture, while sex differences were more prominent in India.

Mar (1971) found male superiority in creativity over females in the study of Arab and American eighth graders. In this study boys performed better on 9 out of 13 scores derived on Torrance Tests of

Creative Thinking.

Indian Studies

Prakash (1969) and Raina (1969) with independent data collected from different parts of the country and about five years apart, found that boys excelled girls on practically all of the verbal creativity tests.

Raina (1969) tried to study the comparative performance of boys and girls on the test of creativity using 180 subjects (90 males and 90 females) of VIII through X classes of higher secondary schools of Ajmer. The results of these study showed that males were more creative than females on the figural tests and on the parts of the verbal form.

Rawat and Agarwal (1977) conducted a study to determine the effects of intelligence, age, sex, community and income groups on creativity. They constructed a test of creative thinking comprising 4 sub-tests; Word Association, Unusual Uses, Plot Titles and Consequences and it was administered to 300, 12-16 year old Indian 8th and 9th graders. Results showed the following: (a) high achievers in intelligence were not necessarily the high achievers in creativity; (b) upto age 13 years boys scored higher than girls, but after 13 years there was a downward trend for boys and an upward trend for girls. At age 16, girl's performance was better than that of the boys; (c) boy's scores on creative thinking were higher than that of the girls in all samples; (d) for boys, caste played no important role in creative thinking, while it affected the girl's scores; (e) occupational community had no impact on role in creative thinking except for the higher income group.

Tara (1981) conducted a study on sex differences in creativity among early adolescents. From schools in Bangalore, 1250 boys and girls of 13-15 years olds were administered the Mehdi's Verbal and Figural Tests of Creativity Thinking. Results showed that males excelled females on measures of verbal fluency, verbal flexibility, figural originality and figural elaboration.

Dharmangadan (1981) conducted a study to determine the effect of sex, age and locale of secondary school pupils on the performance of creativity tests. He administered an adapted version of the Torrance Tests of Creative Thinking to 300 children (12.3-15.5 years of age) from the schools in the Trivandrum. Results showed that (a) boys scored significantly higher than girls; (b) both 14 and 15 year old scored significantly higher than 13 year old; (c) only on verbal tests did, 15 years olds scored higher than 14 year olds and (d) in verbal tests, the urban children scored higher than the rural children.

The study of Tuli (1982) also revealed that boys were significantly more creative than girls in Mathematics.

According to Bhaskara (1986) boys were significantly better than girls on creativity measures. His results were supported by the findings of Prakash (1966), Raina (1960), and Passi, (1972) also.

Shukla and Sharma (1986) studied differences in scientific creativity in 17 males and 13 females in the middle schools of Raipur and Rajnadgaon districts in India. The test of scientific creativity developed by Shukla (1980), which measure fluency, flexibility, originality and global scientific creativity was administered. Results indicated that measures of scientific creativity. The mean scores of boys on all measures of scientific creativity were consistently but insignificantly higher than those of girls.

2. Studies Reporting Girls are Highly Creative

Western Studies

Getzels and Jackson (1962) found that personality dimensions associated with the divergent thinking abilities should provide girls better chances to grow as creative persons but only in respect of semantic content. This is probably due to the fact that the girls tend to keep themselves free from all sense of responsibility likely to occur in different occupations and jobs.

Razik (1964) observed that the females out-ranked males in their creative ability on four out of six tests of creativity. The sample included the students from colleges of Agriculture, Education, Engineering and Applied Arts.

MacGregor and Smith (1965) and Harlow (1967) found that the girls excelled the boys in originality.

Torrance (1967) and his associates found that in he U.S.A after about the age of ten years, the girls consistently performed better than the boys in almost every verbal test of creative thinking.

Orcutt (1968) has given a series of creativity, conformity, and originality tests to 197 children of ages 3, 4 and 5 years. Five year old girls were found to be significantly more conforming than 5 year old boys on this task.

Torrance and Aliotti (1969), with a sample of 10 year old rural Wisconsin children, found that girls expelled in all of he verbal tests and on the figural elaboration test but that boys were superior to girls in figural originality and flexibility. They interpreted this as resulting from greater socio cultural encouragement for boys to be original and divergent with non-verbal concepts and relatively greater social pressures for girls to develop skills that require verbal reinforcement.

The trend of observation, girls are better in creative thinking than boys is also supported by findings of quite a good number of investigations where children from first through sixth grade were involved (MacGregor and Smith, 1965; Ogletree, 1968; Solomon, 1968; Walker, 1969; Cacha, 1971; and Burgess, 1971). In Newlands (1981) experiments, females scored higher than males in creativity tests.

Kershner and Ledger (1985) compared 30 gifted (15 boys and 15 girls, aged 9-11 years) to 30 average IQ children from Toronto Public School on Torrance Tests of Creative Thinking and Thinking Styles. The results showed that sex, IQ and thinking style each had an effect on different dimensions of children's creativity. Girls, irrespective of their IQ level thinking style, scored higher than boys consistently across the seven creativity sub-scales, reaching statistical significance in verbal and figural fluency. Gifted boys and girls, independent of their thinking style than the non-gifted children but only in verbal originality.

Indian Studies

Hussain's (1974) study was on creativity and sex differences. Two groups of boys and girls were formed. Groups I consisted of 100 girls of 10 to 14 years of age, reading in the Muslim University Girl's High School, Aligarh and coming from the upper and middle strata to the society. Group II comprised 100 boys reading in a High School situated in a rural area. Most of them belonged to lower middle class family. Mehdi's Test of Creativity namely Consequences, Unusual Uses, Noval Uses and Elaboration Tests were administered to both the groups. It was found that the creativity score of female group was always higher than male group though the differences were not significant in Consequences, Novel Uses and Elaboration Tests except on Unusual Uses Test.

Gakhar (1974) reported that in Grade X girls scored higher than boys on flexibility.

Singh (1978) suggested that girls scored higher than boys mainly in semantic content. On the figural elaboration the two groups demonstrated performance up to the same level. The girl's group was also able to demonstrate higher level of autonomy in thinking, non-conformity to conventions and less rigidity in belief systems than boys.

Raina (1980) reported a reversal in sex differences in creativity over a 10 year period in India. In 1969, boys in India had shown a consistent superiority on both the verbal and figural creativity. It had shifted on favour of the girls.

Maccoby and Jacklin (1974), and Jarial (1982) found that females students were superior to males in verbal creativity.

In similar investigations, Raina (1971), Goyal (1973) and Sharma (1981) also found that females were significantly superior to males on all the dimensions of creativity, viz., fluency, flexibility and originality.

Chandha and Ghose (1985) found statistically significant difference between males and females on all the components of creativity. The results were in line with the study conducted by Getzels and Jackson (1962), Passi (1972), Brodley (1976) and Chadha (1981) in which they found females scored higher than males on all the four components of creativity.

Asifa (1987) administered Passi Verbal Test of Creativity to a sample of 250 students of IX class (boys-112 and girls-138) of Indore. Girls were found superior to boys in verbal creativity.

3. Studies Reporting No Sex Differences

Western Studies

After reviewing a large number of studies, Maccoby and Jacklin (1974) concluded that no sex differences were found on verbal tests of creativity in pre school and earlier school years, but from about age of seven, girls showed an advantaged in a majority of students. On non-verbal measure no clear trend towards superiority of either sex could be discerned. This observation was substantiated by a number of studies (Olton, 1969; Goyal, 1973 and Panucci, 1978).

Ward (1968) Wallach and Kogan (1965), Gakhar (1974) and Chandha and Sen (1981) also did not did not find any significant sex difference.

Ward and Cox (1974) did not any significant sex difference with respect to either creativity in total or on most of the creative abilities. Similar findings were obtained in the studies of high school children also (Neufield, 1964; Flecther, 1968 and Ogletree, 1968).

Several investigations, involving samples ranging from elementary school children through high school to college students have indicated that there are no sex differences in creativity (Phatak, 1962; Jackson, 1968; Simpkins and Eisenman, 1968; Burns, 1969; Kaltsounis, 1971; Phillips and Torrance, 1971 and Kloss, 1972).

Indian Studies

No significant sex differences were found in three verbal subtests of the Passi test of creativity (Jarial, 1982).

Venkateswara Rao (1987) found that the sex did not effect the creative performance of his subjects.

Asifa (1987) observed that 127 studies were conducted to study sex difference in creativity during the period of 1905 to 1981. Out of which 42 were in India, rest abroad and 39.37 per cent of these studies found superiority of female over male in verbal and non-verbal creativity, whereas 25.19 per cent found males superior to females in creativity. The remaining 35.43 per cent found no significant difference in the creativity of males and females.

Studies on Age and Sex Difference and Field Dependence/Independence Cognitive Styles

Western Studies

Miller (1953), Gump (1955), Zuckman (1957), Bieri, Bradburn and Galinsky (1958), Young (1959) and Witkin, et al (1962) found that males were more field independent and more articulated in their approach to certain perceptual tasks than females.

Consistent sex differences have repeatedly been found in the field dependence dimension. Boys and men tend to be more field independent than girls and women, small but consistent sex difference were observed in the Embedded Figures Test and in other tests of field dependence, both in the United States and a number of Western European Countries (e.g., Witt, 1955; Bennett, 1956; Franks, 1956), and in Hong Kong (Goodnow, unpublished study), Japan (Kato, 1965), Israel (Rothman, unpublished study), Sierra Leone, Africa (Dawson, 1967) and Nigeria (Okonji, 1969) as well. The Weight of the present evidence indicates that sex differences may not be present before the age of eight or in geriatric groups.

Crandall and Sinkeldam (1964) found that older and more intelligent children exhibited more perceptual-independence than younger and less intelligent ones, and non-significant trend was found for boys to perform more proficiently on the Embedded Figures Test than girls.

Witkin, Goodenough and Karp (1967) found there are clear age related changes in field dependence over the life span. Developmental curves for the Embedded Figures Test Rod-and-Frame Test and Body Adjustment Test, Covering the 8 to 24 year period, showed a marked, continuous increase in field independence between 8 and about 15 years, although in this period the rate of change showed down with increasing age. After age of 15 years the developmental curves showed a levelling off and approach a plateau in the period of young adulthood.

In the data discussed by Coates (1974), the sex difference favouring females was most pronounced at 5 years and had begun to reverse by 6 years. This is consistent with the Children's Embedded Figures Test standardization data for children aged 7-12 years, where man differences , although not statistically significant, nevertheless favoured males (Karp and Konstadt, 1971).

Kogan (1976) reported that sex differences on field independence/dependence in selective college samples are frequently not found. In short there is a relatively brief period early in the life span - where female superiority in disembedding skill has been clearly demonstrated.

Huss and Kayson (1985) investigated the effects of age and sex on speed of finding imbedded figures. The sample consisted of 20 male and 20 female students. Ten of each sex was in grade 3 or 4 and 10 of each sex was in grade 11 or 12. Each subject was given 3 pairs of figures and told to find the simple figure that was embedded in more complex figure. Results showed that sex and age were significant. Boys found the hidden figures faster that girls, and older subjects were faster than younger ones.

Drouin, Talbot, and Goulet (1986) investigated the field dependence/independence of 77 female and 115 male French Canadian University athletes by means of the Embedded figures Test. There were no significant difference by age, level of competition or sports.

Bill (1987) conducted a study on examination of developmental trends in fields dependence among age groups of 13 or 21 years of age. The subjects were 120, 13-15 year olds, 120, 16-18 year olds and 120, 19-21 year olds. They were tested on a rod and frame apparatus. Result showed that 16-18 year olds were more field independent. Developmental trends indicated decreased field dependence into late adolescence and increased field dependence in early adulthood.

Studies on Age and Sex Differences and Reflection/Impulsivity Cognitive Style

Western Studies

Very few studies are reported on reflection/ impulsivity cognitive style with regard to age and sex differences. Children typically become more reflective with age. The increase response times and decrease errors on the Matching Familiar Figures Test a finding confirmed both by cross-sectional and longitudinal studies (Ault, 1973; Campbell and Douglas, 1972; Fancher, 1969; Kagan, 1965; Ward, 1973). In addition, the negative correlation between response time and errors tends to become larger with age . This relationship is considerately less robust in pre school age than in school age children.

Wright (1973) who administered the Kogan's Reflection/Impulsivity Scale for pre school children to a cross-sectional sample of 3, 4 and 6 year old middle class children, found that the relationship between response time and errors increased with age for boys but decreased with age for girls.

Salkind and Wright (1977) had given a note on the developmental nature of reflection/impulsivity. The hypothesis that children become more reflective as they get older was tested using the norms developed for the Matching Familiar Figures Test. Results showed that for both sexes up through age 10 years, a decrease in errors and an increase in latency were found. After that age errors stabilized and latency decreased. Correlations between errors and latency also peaked at age 10 (lowest for the youngest and oldest groups).

INFLUENCE OF PSYCHOLOGICAL FACTORS ON CREATIVITY AND COGNITIVE STYLES

Studies on Personality and Creativity

An important aspect of research on creativity has been the study of it's relationship with personality characteristics. It is a common belief that creative persons are different from others in the sense that they have unique personality traits. The personality includes the overall traits of an individual.

Western Studies

From interviews with a fourth grade group of creative children and a control group of comparable IQ and age, Weisberg and Springer (1961) concluded that the creative children significantly demonstrated a stronger self-image, greater ease of early recall, humour, availability of oedipal anxiety, and uneven ego development.

Torrance (1962) found that highly creative children are not always well-rounded individuals. An imaginative or inventive child who is an expert in solving problems and developing fantastic ideas may have reading or writing difficulties. Their visuals abilities may be below some of their other abilities or they may be inferior to their fellows in size and strength. They are also likely to have physical defects or impairments.

Barron's (1963) study analyzed personality attributes of creative individuals. The attributes are based on 76 descriptive statements of personal functioning sorted on a 9 point scale and 300 item checklist of adjectives checked simply as characteristic or non-characteristic of a creative person. It was found that creative individuals are seen as intelligent, interesting, and imaginative people-quick, flexible and perceptive, socially effective and personally dominant.

Taylor's (1964) study reveals three major characteristic of creative people. They are (1) intellectual, originality, flexibility, sensitivity, memory and evaluation; (2) motivational interest, curiosity, likes to play with others, challenged by problems, tolerate uncertainty, persistent and committed to his or her work; and (3) personality (independent, more inclined to risk, more resourceful and adventurous).

Cashdon and Welsh (1966) showed that the high creative adolescent emerged as an independent, non-conforming individual who seeks change in his environment and whose interpersonal relationship is open and active.

Parloff and Datta (1966) explored the personality characteristics of male high school entrants in the Westing House Science Talent Search. On the basis of their judged creativity and potential creativity, the sample of 537 students were divided into high, moderate and low groups of potential creativity. Although the groups did not differ significantly in terms of age, IQ science aptitude socio economic status, and the inactness in the family, there were statistically significant differences in the personality characteristics as determined by personality tests. They state: Group I was significantly higher than Group III on the capacity for status, more ambitious and driving, more independent autonomous and self-reliant male more efficient use of their intelligence and were more perceptive. Group II in contrast to group I had less a feeling or well-being, less control, more impulsive, less concerned about impressions on others and less efficient in the use of intelligence.

Kurtzman (1967) compared three groups of adolescents with different levels of creativity to determine it they differed with respect to personality characteristics - peer acceptance and attitude toward schools. The result indicate that creative students tend to be move adventurous, extroverted and self-confident. They also have a less favourable attitude towards schools. In terms of peer acceptance, sex appeared to be an important factor. Higher creative boys received greater accepted by their classmates.

Iwata (1968) studied relationship of creativity with intelligence and personality variables and found that in the upper half of an intelligence test but in the lower half on the creativity test, the subjects were more independent introverted and dominant but less sociable than those in the lower half in intelligence but in the upper half in the creativity. Those high on creativity test were relatively more extroverted and less neurotic.

White (1968) examined two major 2nd order factor (Anxiety and Introversion-Extroversion) from the Cattell's 16 PF and measures of divergent ability as measured by Wilson's Alternate Uses Test and Christensen's Consequences Test found that the persons having relatively low level of anxiety performed significantly better on divergent thinking tasks. Extroverts were found to have high scores on divergent thinking, ability of flexibility, fluency, and originality than the introverts.

Torrance's (1969) study revealed more creative group was found to have significantly higher scores than the less creative group on the scales for achievement, affiliation, conjunctivity, ego energy, exhibition, reflectiveness, and understanding.

Barron (1969) summarized the studies of creative mathematicians, scientists, writers, architects and business managers, and found that in addition to being flexible, curious and original, they were individualistic, non-conforming, unsociable, low in impulse traits might have enabled the highly creative children to preserve and to develop their scientific creativity.

Khire (1971) studied creativity in relation to intelligence and personality factors. A battery of creativity tests was developed and Raven's Advanced Progressive Matrices was used to measure creativity an intelligence. The cognitive and non-cognitive measures included the scores on the Bennet's Mechanical Comprehension Test, school marks, interests regarding academic subjects, games, hobbies, students rating of peers and teachers and the scores on the Bernreuter's Personality Inventory for the upper extreme group-first 25 on creativity and first 25 on intelligence. Some of the important findings were (i) the chosen variables of creativity (abilities of fluency, flexibility, originality and elaboration) remained closer to each other and at the same time farther from intelligence; (ii) creativity had lower correlation with aptitude of mechanical comprehension and higher with scholastic performance as compared to intelligence and (iii) high quality of academic performance was related with high creativity.

Komarik (1972) studied the relations between creativity and other measures of personality namely, intelligence and Eysenck's orthogonal factors. A significant positive correlation was found between creativity and neuroticism, while no significant relationship was found between creativity and extroversion or creativity and intelligence. It was suggested that L-score of E.P.I may be an indicator of social conformity which is an impediment to creativity.

Singer and Rummo (1973) reported that teachers were found to rate highly creative children as less autonomous, less persistent in doing tasks, and less accepting of responsibility.

Hassan and Akbar (1973) in their study on ideal and perceived self-concept of high and low creative students found that high creative group students were less satisfied with the qualities they perceived to have and they wished to be self - confident and systematic than the low creative group.

Besides, personality correlates of 16 PF test with creativity, several other personality tests have also been investigated in reaction to creative individuals. Thus, Phillips (1973) studied the relationship between creativity performance and personality profiles by median split on the Torrance Test of Creative Thinking into high and low creative groups. He compared two groups on the Omnibus Personality Inventory and found that the high and the low creative subjects differed significantly in terms of some personality factors and the way in which they perceived themselves. It was also observed that within each group significant relationships were found between personality profiles and self perceptions.

Payne, Helpin, Ellett, and Dale (1975) studied personality correlates of creativeness in two groups - academically and artistically gifted youths and obtained multiple correlations between sub-scales of the 16 PF and Torrance and Khatana's what kind of person are you? Inventory-a measure of creative personality characteristics. The 5 most significant scales yielded multiple correlations of 0.56 for the academic group 0.71 for the artistic group, and 0.61 for the combined groups. The self report characteristics of shrewd and reserved were descriptive of the academic and combined talented groups. The scale of self-sufficient, sensitivity and casualness were descriptive of artistic group.

Wolhers (1976) observed two personality characteristics - complexity and integration, to play an important role in creative individuals. The creative personality was further described as unbalanced, differentiated, independent, tolerant with respect to ambiguity, and permissive.

Indian Studies

Bhattacharya (1961) conducted a survey of 20 well known painters in India, to know their personality and found that the subjects were introverted since childhood. He isolated the following psychological qualities, intelligence, constructive capacity, relative ideas of form and depth, confidence, sociability, and spontaneous reaction to stimulation. The survey also suggested that the painter's sex differences and religion played no significant role in his/her creative activity.

Raychaudhuri (1961) using projective techniques and clinical ratings found the artists to have among others, a high degree of sensitivity and on ability of playful "prelogical" thinking. In another study, he found musicians to have sufficient emotional breadth and tendency to seek intimate interpersonal relationship. They appeared to meet the frustration and anxiety, including situation, as a challenge.

Raina (1968) in his Doctoral study on some personality correlates in Indian students found the highly creative, high school students exhibiting greater achievement, autonomy, dominance, change and endurance than the low creative students.

Goyal (1969) studied personality traits of reactive children at the middle school stage of Patiala district in Punjab. Using his own valid and reliable tests of creativity developed on the lines of Torrance, he concluded that the creative pupils at the middle school stage possessed a higher level of energy; they rejected suppression foot the control of impulses; they were more of introverts and more independent in both thought and action; had open minds; could tolerate ambiguity and entertained opposing values.

Ahmad (1969) tried to study the personality differences among high and low creativity girls. A 94 items test of personality from Sen's Personality Trait Inventor, including six areas of personality, viz., (i) activity (ii) attempt at moral values, (iii) dominance, (iv) depressive tendency, (v) emotional instability, and (vi) introversion, was administered to the two groups of creative and non-creative girls. The obtained results indicated that the two groups did not differ significantly on any of the personality traits except dominance. The originals or the creatives were more dominant than the unoriginals or the low creatives.

Srichandra (1970) made a socio-psychological study of frustration among Indian scientists. His sample consisted of a large number of individuals drawn from Universities and Research Institutes in India. He has listed a number of sources of frustration as found in these scientists. These included incongruence in the image of self and that of authority, perception of incompetence of authority, discrepancy between achievement and aspiration, feelings of incompetence and insecurity among others.

Passi (1972) conducted an exploratory study of creativity and it's relationship with intelligence and achievement in school subjects at higher secondary stage. The sample consisted of 600 higher secondary boys and girls of rural and urban areas of the Punjab, Haryana and Chandigarh. Different tools, namely questionnaire for personal data, the Things Done of Your Own, the Raven's Standard Progressive Matrices Test, the Jalota's Group Test of General Mental Ability, Scholastic achievement from school records and the Passi's Test of Creativity were used to collect data. The results reported that the scores of the criterion variable of scholastic achievement were found to be significantly influenced by the major effects of sex, residence, grade, creativity and intelligence as well as the interactional effects of sex x residence x grade.

Recently in a study employing Wallach-Kogan tests for measuring creativity. Parmesh (1972) concluded that the high creative individuals were neither significantly more or less introverted than the low creative individuals. The high creative individuals were not significantly different from the low creative individuals in the level of anxiety and neuroticism. The high creatives were significantly high in ego - strength than the low creative individuals. The high creatives differed significantly from the low creatives on theoretical and aesthetic values.

Joshi (1974) studied creativity and some personality traits of the intellectually gifted high school students. The sample consisted of 935 gifted pupils from standards VII to XII of 23 secondary schools of Ahmedabad, Baroda, Karia, Panchmahals and Surat. They were administered Torrance Creativity Test and Cattell's 16 PF Test. Their annual examination marks were treated as achievement scores. It was found that giftedness was an effective contributor, to creative scores. Age was an important correlate of creativity at 15 years age-level. Giftedness contributed to emotional maturity in boys and to personality factor B in all cases. There was a low positive creativity and creativity and achievement in all school subjects except English.

Gopal (1975) investigated the personality variables of creative and non-creativity science and engineering students. The findings were: creative science and engineering students were found to be more reserved, emotionally stable, assertive, expedient, venturesome, self-sufficient and relaxed than the counterpart group.

Gakhar (1975) studied intellectual and personality correlates of creativity. The sample was 730 girls from IX, X and XI of high schools in urban areas of Punjab. Torrance Test of Creative Thinking form A and figural form A, the Group Test of General Mental Ability by Jalota and Singh. The California Psychological Inventory and the Bernreuter Personality Inventory were administered. The main findings were that both creativity and intelligence were two distinguishable modes of the same intelligence functioning, yet at the same time they were not distinctly independent of each other out of 24 personality traits chosen in the study fifteen were correlated positively with verbal creativity while 18 were correlated positively with non-verbal creativity. There was a consistent increase in the mean scores from grades IX to XI on all the measures until about age of 15 years, though some non-verbal creativity was found to develop even beyond this age.

Kumar (1975) has shown that on difficult, insightful problem solving tasks, introverts performed significantly better than extroverts on both the number of trails and time taken.

Passi and Lalitha (1975) conducted a factorial study of creativity, intelligence, and self-concept of adolescents. The sample consisted of 68 boys and 49 girls of grade X from three English Medium High Schools of Baroda city. The Passi's (1973) Test of Creativity (PTC) was used to measure general intelligence. The personality word list (Deo, 1963) used to measure perceived self-concept. The findings of the study were as follows:

1. **Varimax factor I**—Most of these factor loadings are on the dimension of positive self-concept.
2. **Varimax factor II**—This factor involving mental functions can be named as verbal creativity. Verbal creativity has significant loading on variables namely verbal fluency, flexibility, originality and claboration.
3. **Varimax factor III**—This factor is heavily loaded by negative components of self-concept.
4. **Varimax factor IV**—Peculiar pattern of factor loadings, such as age, increase intelligence and scholastic achievement amongst adolescents decrease.
5. **Varimax factor V**—The dimensions of negative self concept

have positive loadings and those of positive self-concept, negative loadings.

6. **Varimax factor VI**—This factor has been named as self-concept aesthetic. The other dimensions of self-concept namely intelligence, character, social and emotional adjustment could not be represented by respective factors.

Nair (1975) conducted a study to solve the problem of identification of the creative pupils in the class room by simple observation of the adjustive nature of their personality. The positive adjustment variables subjected to experimentation were self-reliance, sense of personal worth, sense of personal freedom, feeling of belonging, freedom from withdrawing tendencies, freedom from nervous symptoms social standards, social skills freedom from anti-social tendencies, family relations, school relations and community relations. The only negative adjustment variable under experimentation was anxiety. The test of creative thinking developed by the researcher included fluency, flexibility, originality, elaboration, sensitivity to problems and redefinition. The study indicated that the creative pupils were found to differ from the non-creative pupils in respect of the adjustment variables, viz., covert sense of personal freedom, freedom from withdrawing tendencies, freedom from anti-social tendencies, school relations, community relations and anxiety to a high degree. In respect of variables comprising self-reliance, sense of personal worth, feeling of belonging, freedom from nervous symptoms, social standards and social skills, the creative pupils differed from the non-creative to a comparatively lesser degree. The profile of the adjustive traits of the creative pupils was found to differ significantly from that of the non-creative pupils. The non-creative pupils exhibited the highest degree of the feeling or anxiety whereas the creative pupils the lowest degree. The creative pupils were better adjusted than the non-creative pupils, personally as well as socially.

Jawa (1976) observed that personality, perceptual, environmental and structural factors interacted to determine creative behaviour amongst students of secondary schools.

Patel (1976) studied personality syndromes of people who are high on each of five creativity dimensions, using Torrance Test of Creative Thinking and a Biographical Inventory form alongwith the 16 PF test and found that those with a high profile on all creativity variables were venturesome, placid, self confident and emotionally stable, while those low on all creative variables were shy.

Paramesh and Narayana (1976) studied the effect of creativity and intelligence on temperament. Ninety three adult graduates employed permanently in a large firm in Madras were taken for the study. The age of the subjects ranged from 23 to 30 years. The Wallach and Kogan (1965) Visual Creativity Instruments, Raven's (1960) Standard Progressive Matrices and Thurstone's Temperament Schedule were administered to the subjects in group form. The results revealed that creativity seems to subdue sociability trait at lower level of intelligence. Creativity seems to subdue active trait at lower levels of intelligence while contributing to the same at higher level of intelligence. Low creative high intelligence group is highest on active trait.

Babu (1977) conducted a comparative study of the personality factors of High Intelligence - High Creative (HI-HC) thinkers and High Intelligence—Low Creative (HI-LC) thinkers in secondary schools in Kerala. Two tests of intelligence—one verbal and other non-verbal and a standardized creativity test in Malayalam was administered. The sample was of 128 HI-HC subjects and 159 HI-LC subjects. The 2 groups were compared on 14 personality variables. It was found that (i) among 14 variables, 8 variables viz., self-reliance, withdrawing tendencies nervous symplons, social standards, anti-social tendencies family relations, school relations and general anxiety discriminated significantly between the two groups; (ii) factors identified for HI-HC group were (a) Non-anxious Disposition (b) Group Adjustment, (c) Individual Adjustment, (d) Social Conformity, (e) Performance Anxiety, (f) Free Orientation, (iii) Factors identified for the HI-LC group were (a) Self-Adjustment, (e) Social Disposition, (f) Total Adjustment; (iv) it was indicated that dissimilarity of factor patterns for HI-HC was because of the presence of 2 factors in each group (Social Conformity and Freedom Orientation for the HI-LC group and Social Disposition and Total Adjustment for the HI-LC group) for which comparable factors did not exist in the other group .

Chauhan's (1977) study on second stratum personality factors, sex and age (adolescence) as correlates of originality. Two hundred and forty 17-21 year old Indian University students showed that (a) originality develops consistently through late adolescence, with adjustment and introversion as negative and positive correlates respectively, and (b) the characteristics of "alert poise" and "being subdued" appear to develop relative to the growth or originality, with males conforming better to this model in mind adolescence and females better in late-adolescence.

Gakhar (1975) and Gupta (1977) found that highly creative individuals were found to possess higher self-concepts and high self-acceptance both of which were conducive to better adjustment and positive mental health.

Nair and Babu (1977) of Kerala University in their factor analytical study of personality variables related to high and low creative thinkers found three factors which characterize the creative group. These were social adequacy feeling, school inadequacy feeling and personal inadequacy feeling.

Mehdi (1977) conducted a correlational study of creativity, intelligence and achievement. Two hundred and fifty nine boys studying in classes 7th and 8th of an urban intermediate college of Aligarh and 200 boys studying in three rural schools of Azamgarh district in U.P formed the sample of the study. The age range of pupils was 12-13 years plus. Creativity was measured by verbal and non-verbal tests of creative thinking prepared by the author (1969-74). General intelligence was measured by a verbal and non-verbal test of general intelligence. ,The annual examination marks represented the school achievement of pupils. In the urban sample, intelligence and creativity are slightly negatively correlated, in he rural sample, they show significantly positive correlations and creativity and school achievement also significantly correlated.

Mallapa and Upadhyaya (1977) have shown that both high and low creative groups are significantly different on factor B, H, Q_2, Q_3 and Q_4 of 16 PF.

Kumar (1978) studied creative functioning in relation to personality structure, value orientation and achievement motivation. Ninety six high and low creative class IX science students of Muzaffar Nagar were given the Torrance Tests of Creative Thinking, Jalota's Test of General Mental Ability and a Hindi version of Eysenck's Introversion-Extroversion Measure. A sentence Completion Test to measure achievement motivation, and a Hindi version of the Allport-Vernon-Lindzey study of values, and were more highly motivated towards achievement.

Asha (1978) conducted a study to find out whether (i) highly creative children differed significantly from their less creative peers in different areas of adjustment such as home, health, social and school adjustments, (ii) highly creative children differed significantly from their less creative peers in adjustment to the problems of stemming from the situation in which they found themselves, and (iii) whether better adjusted children differed from their maladjusted peers in creative performance. The sample comprised 1100 students of standard X drawn from twenty-four high schools in Trivandrum district in Kerala, giving proportional representation to the sex and location and the type of school. The findings of the study indicated that none of the groups classified on the basis of creativity showed significant difference in health, social and school adjustment areas for the boys and girls. Again, it was found that three creative groups among the boys showed significant differences in emotional adjustment. Only two sub-groups (high and moderately creative groups) of boys showed significant difference in low adjustment. Boys and girls differed significantly in adjustment to situations that are assumed to creative problems for creative children. The better adjusted and maladjusted group within each area of adjustment differed only in certain tasks of creativity and these tasks differed for each areas of adjustment. When classified on the basis of problems concerning personality characteristics of creative children, the better adjusted and the maladjusted groups of boys differed in one task of creativity (similarities) and the moderately adjusted and maladjusted girls differed on one task (pattern meaning).

Bhattacharya (1978) studied the interaction of personality and creativity. The sample consisted of 410 male students of classes IX and XI. The findings of the study revealed that there was no interaction of creativity and the fourteen personality factors of High School Personality Questionnaire on the achievement of students of classes IX and X. Factor C, G, H, Q_4 and creativity interacted to affect the intelligence of those in classes IX and XI levels of personality factors did not affect intelligence. Levels of creativity did not affect the intelligence of the students. Levels of any of the fourteen personality factors did not affect the achievement of class XI pupils. Verbal elaboration had a significant positive relationship with composite creativity, fluency, flexibility and originality. Comparability had significant positive relationship positive relationship with creativity and its two components-flexibility and originality. Literary quantitative production was significantly and positively related to composite creativity and all it's components-fluency, flexibility and originality. The high creative secondary and higher secondary students were more warm-heard, more outgoing, more intelligent, less excitable and more adventurous than the low creative secondary students. The low creative secondary students were assertive and aggressive with weaker superego strength, whereas the low creative higher secondary students were conforming, dependent, shy, withdrawing and quick in seeing dangers.

Singh (1978) examined the divergent thinking abilities and creative personality dimensions of bright adolescent boys and girls. One hundred and fifty eight boys and 162 girls were given 17 tests and scales. Results showed that girls had higher levels than boys in word association, ideational and expressional fluency, spontaneous flexibility and originality, autonomy in thinking, non-conformity to conventions and less rigidity in their belief systems.

Jhag (1979) undertook a study of personality correlates of creative children studying science subjects. A sample of 700 higher secondary school students of fifteen plus, drawn from the Bhopal division of Madhya Pradesh. It revealed that scientific creativity was normally distributed. The urban students were superior to the semi-urban, in scientific creativity. The creative and non-creative did not differ significantly on personality factor (reserved vs outgoing). The male and female subjects had more or less similar personality styles in respect of the reserved Vs outgoing trait. Students belonging to the urban and semi-urban background did not differ significantly in personality styles, particularly on the reserved vs. outgoing trait. There was significant contribution of scientific creativity to the variance of factor B (concrete thinking vs abstract thinking). Creative students were significantly better in abstract thinking, emotional stability, independence, self-sufficiency, self-concept and intelligence and were more venturesome, relaxed, controlled and doubting. The creative boys were adventurous, self-assured, placid, secure complacent and serene while the creative girls were shy, timid, restrained and sensitive to threat, guilt-prone, apprehensive, self-reproaching, insecure and worrying. There was no difference in the pattern of personality correlates of creative children from the urban and semi-urban areas. The semi-urban students were more shy, restrained, different and timid than their urban counterparts. The semi-urban boys were more rule bound venturesome, socially old, precise and self disciplined than the urban boys. The urban girls were more rule-bound, assertive and socially precise than the semi-urban girls. There was no significant difference in the achievement of the high creative and high intelligent groups.

Jairal and Sharma (1980) examined the effects and interactions of intelligence and personality on fluency, flexibility, originality and total creativity of 55 urban high school students. Subjects were administered the Passi Test of Creativity, Maudsley Personality Inventory and Group General Mental Ability Test and were divided into high and low intelligence on fluency, originality and total creativity of subjects. Introverts and extroverts differed among themselves on originality.

Muddu (1980) made an attempt to measure the degree of creativity among school-going students in Andhra Pradesh and also tried to investigate the relationship of certain variables to creativity. The sample consisted of 474 boys drawn from various high school of Hyderabad and Secunderabad. Cluster and multi-stage sampling technique was adopted in the selection of sample. The study indicated that the high creative group was found to be negatively correlated (r = 0.096) with intelligence, weaker super-ago strength, emotional indulgence, high strength of self-sentiment and low tension were positively and significantly correlated with intelligence. Creativity was found to be having highly significant relationship with fluency (r=0.777). Relationship between intelligence and fluency (r=124) , flexibility (r=114) and originality (r=0.125) were positively and significant. Personality characteristics of the high creative groups totally differed from those of the low creative groups. The high as well as the low creative groups did not show any significant correlation with intelligence. Low creative boys are more fluent than the high creative boys. There was no significant relationship between the high intelligent group and the low creative group and between the high creative group and the intelligent group. The creative children were controlled, striving to get acceptance and approval, ethically standard, ambitious to do well, concerned with social images, considerate of other foresighted, conscientious, relaxed, unfrustrated and composed. Personality characteristics of the low creative boys were temperamental and resurgent. The high creative boys were emotionally controlled and self-assured.

Creativity within the framework of personalogical context was studied by Gakhar and Joshi (1980). A total of 730 subjects were drawn from IX, X and XI grades from Government school of Punjab State.

Torrance Tests of Creative Thinking (1966) , Gough's California Psychological Inventory (1964) and the Bernreuter Personality Inventory (1935) were administered to measure creativity and personality. Results indicated that the traits of personality in general did not exhibit a consistent picture of correlation with all the creative ability measures on verbal and figural creativity. Within the separate domains of verbal and figural creative abilities, the association of personality traits was not consistent for all creative abilities (fluency, flexibility, originality and elaboration).

Sharma (1981) studied the intrinsic value structures and creativity among higher secondary school girls. Administered 3 Verbal Creativity Tests (Utility, Word Association and Plot Titles) and an Intrinsic Values Inventory assessing altruism, productivity, independence, intellectual stimulation, and aesthetics to 100 Indian females. Product moment correlation showed that of the creativity scores fluency was not related to any intrinsic value, flexibility was positively related to intellectual stimulation, and originality was positively related to both independence and intellectual stimulation and negatively to altruism. Total creativity was marginally related to intellectual stimulation.

The nature and extent of the relationship between creativity and adjustment was studied by Singh (1981). The sample was 600 male student of high school classes from Agra city. Mehdi's (1973) Verbal Test of Creativity Thinking and Adjustment Inventory for school students prepared by Sinha and Sigh (1972) were administered. Positive correlations were seen between creativity and the different areas of adjustment except in the case of emotional. But, their strength was low. High creative groups better adjusted than average and low creative groups. High and low creative groups differed in emotional and educational areas of adjustment.

Singh (1981) studied creativity as function of adjustment, frustration and level of aspiration. The sample was 135 high school students who were high, moderate or low on all three variables. As predicted, adjustment, frustration, and aspiration had no effect on creativity either alone or interaction with one another.

Kishore (1981) made an attempt to explore creativity in preadolescent children at secondary school stage. The sample consisted of 965 students of classes VI to X of a single school. The tools used were the

Creativity Tests developed by the investigator, General Intelligence Test and High School Personality Questionnaire. Scores for creativity and personality characteristic of various grades indicated that during classes VI to VIII divergent traits of personality, viz., outgoing, more intelligent, emotionally, stable, excitable, assertive, happy-go-lucky, venturesome, doubting, self-sufficient, expedient, tough-minded, placid, indisciplined and relaxed were found consistently associated with all the creativity measures. In the latter classes IX, X convergent personality traits different from those listed above (except intelligence) were found highly correlated with all the creativity measures.

Bali (1981) investigated common personality factors of highly creative persons in different field, viz., poetry, painting, science and music. The sample consisted of 20 persons who had been rewarded or recognised in their fields. They were administered Cattell's 16 PF Test Form-A, Their scores on 16 PF in terms of O and C and also trait-wise constituted the basic data of the study. Q-technique of factor analysis was used to analyze the data. Six factors were identified as emotional, sensitivity, ego-deal, introversion, creative mood and social will. Longitudinal interpretations of factors matrix revealed: (i) Poets possessed factors like emotional sensitivity, creative mood and social will; (ii) painters profile consisted of common factors like emotional sensitivity and creative mood; (iii) scientists profile consisted of common factors of ego-ideal, emotional introversion and social will; and (iv) musicians profile showed factors of ego-ideal and social will.

Chandha and Sen (1981) conducted a study to see the relationship between creativity, personality and vocational interest of twelfth grade students of Delhi School. Administered the Thurstone Interest Schedule, Torrance Tests of Creative Thinking and Maudsley Personality Inventory to 55 male and 61 female students. It was found that extroversion was related to creativity for male only and females tended to have higher extroversion scores than males. Creativity had significant positive relation with business and executive interests, and a negative relation with computation.

Agarwal and Bohra (1982) studied the personality pattern of high and low creative children. Eighty children of eighth standard of a Middle School of Jodhpur city were administered Verbal Test of Creativity Thinking (Mehdi, 1973). On the basis of scores on this test, twenty children were placed into high creative group and twenty into low creative group. The two groups were administered Cattell's Junior-

Senior High School Personality Questionnaire (Indian modification by Kapoor and Malhotra, 1975). Results showed the significant difference in the two groups of factors A, B, C, E, and H.

Rastogi and Nathawt (1982) conducted a study to see the relationship between creativity and mental health in male and female adolescents. A sample of 50 boys and 50 girls from 9th, 10th, and 11th standards of the Central School at Jaipur, Maslow's Security - Insecurity (S-I) Inventory and Wallach and Kogan Test of Creativity (1965) were used to assess the mental health and creativity respectively. It was found that emotionally secure adolescents had high creativity level as compared to their emotionally insecure counterparts. Sex and emotional security - insecurity level of the subjects have no interactional effect on creativity.

Singh (1982) conducted a study to find out the relationship between creativity, intelligence and socio-economic status. The sample for the study consisted of 400 rural and 400 urban high school students drawn from sixteen Intermediate Colleges in Varanasi and Faizabad division. The study depicted that the mean intelligence score of the urban students was significantly higher than that of the rural students. In general, the socio economic status of the urban students was higher than that of the students from rural areas. The mean creativity score of the urban students was higher than that of the students from rural areas. The mean creativity score of science students was higher than that of arts students.

Rai (1982) conducted a study to identify creative and non-creative students. He also tried to find out the difference in problem-solving ability between the creative and non-creative students. The sample of the study consisted of 200 students from two secondary schools of Patna. The main finding of the study was that the creative and non-creative groups differed significantly in their problem-solving ability. There was thus need for more tasks to the creative students after they were identified.

Venkata Rami Reddy and Balakrishna Reddy (1983) studied creativity and intelligence. A creativity test battery consisting of 10 sub-tests, and the Raven's Standard Progressive Matrices were administered to 70 High School student selected by Multistage Stratified Random Sampling procedure. The total creativity score and mental ability were found to be significantly correlated except in the case of

Impossibilities Test. But, the correlation was insignificant in the high ability sub-group.

Goyal's (1984) study aimed to isolate the personality characteristics that differentiate the high creative student teachers from the low creative. The Verbal and Non-verbal Form A of the Torrance Tests of Creative Thinking and the 16 PF were administered, after due adaptation, to 500 B.ED. students randomly selected from five teacher training colleges of Punjab. The criterion group were identified on the basis of ± 1 SD from the mean. The t-test results indicated that intelligence (factor B) was the only factor which discriminated between the high and low creatives, the high creative being higher on it.

Arora (1985) studied 800 college students in different streams of professional courses completed personality tests. Finding indicate that personality adjustment was inversely correlated with self-concept and creative potential, but was positively correlated with level of aspiration, creative potential was inversely correlated with self-concept.

Helode (1986) administered a diagnostic test for extroversion-introversion to 90 male and 115 female Indian adolescents. As hypothesized , males exhibited a greater degree of the Expressed Characteristics (ECS) of the creative person compared to females, extroversion showed a significant negative relationship with ECs of creative persons. Introverted males had a higher level of ECs than extroverted females.

Saxena and Sharma (1986) studied the relationship between creative functioning and adjustment patterns among male high school students (aged 14-16 years) in India. Among 80 randomly selected subjects, 20 were identified as high creative and 20 low creative on the Verbal Test of Creative Thinking by Mehdi (1973). These subjects completed the High School Adjustment Inventory by Sinha and Singh (1971). Scores were obtained for emotional, social, educational, and overall adjustment. In comparison to low creatives, high creatives scored higher on emotional and social adjustment but lower on educational and overall adjustment.

Matthews (1986) tested the effects on intelligence and creative test performance of 2 sixteen Personality Factor Questinnaire (16 PF), primary anxiety traits and general mood and activation components of state anxiety Two attentional theories of the deleterious effects of anxiety on performance were also tested. Subjects were 80 male university students. Trait and state components of anxiety appeared to affect creativity test performance independently. Intelligence test performance was insensitive to anxiety variables. The O (worry) anxiety primary factor was significantly negatively correlated with creativity test performance but the unique variance of the Q_4 (emotionality) factor was associated with higher levels of performance.

An empirical investigation of creativity, ego-strength and extroversion was conducted by Kundu (1986). The subjects in this study comprised XI grade students of Arts and Natural Science from Central Schools in Delhi. For measuring creativity, Torrance Tests of Creative Thinking was administered. For measuring extroversion, neuroticism, and psychoticism, Eysenck Personality Questionnaire was employed. For measuring ego-strength, Bender Gestalt's Test was used. The findings are as follows: (1) introverts are more creative than extroverts; (2) creativity is positively and highly related with ego-strength; (3) science students are more creative than arts students; (4) creativity is negatively and highly related with psychoticism; (5) the relationship between creativity and extroversion is curvilinear; (6) dysthemics are more creative than hysterics; (7) introverts with higher ego-strength are more creative than extroverts with higher ego-strength.

Recently, kumar and Kapila (1987) have reported that introverts were significantly superior to extroverts on insightful problem irrespective of sex and scores on Bem sex-role Inventory.

Sumangala (1987) studied the relationship between Social adjustment and creativity with 262 secondary school pupils (107 boys and 155 girls) of standard IX selected from 12 schools in Kerala and concluded that the relationship between creativity and social adjustment could be explained by assessing creative activities that are performed by subjects to communicate with others and to gain acceptance. It may be this communication ability that causes the relationship between creativity and social adjustments.

Kumar and Kumari (1988) conducted a study on problem-solving as a function of creativity and personality. A selected sample of 48 students of Punjab Agricultural University, Ludhiana, was equally divided into two creative (high and low) group and two personality (extroversion and introversion) groups. The subjects were given the two problems as anagram tasks and candle-stick task. Performance in anagram task was assessed in terms of a number of correct solutions in 10 minutes, where as, in candle-stick task, the index of performances was the time taken to solve the problem. The data were analyzed by ANOVA. The findings are: (1) the high creative group and introverts are superior to their respective counterparts. The F-ratios in both the cases are significnt ($P < 0.01$); (2) a significant creativity X personality interaction on anagram task reveals that high creativity boosts the performance of extroveted subjects, share as the introverts remain steady and superior under both the conditions of creativity.

Studies on Personality and Field Dependence/Independence Cognitive Style

Western Studies

Since the inception of the field dependence/independence dimension (Witkin, et al., 1954), it has been assumed individuals positions along the field-dependence/independence continuum are related to a number of personality and behavioural correlates (Long, 1974; O' Leary, et al., 1980).

Woerner and Levine (1950) found significant relationship between field dependence measures and IQ scores on the Wechsler Intelligence Scale for Children (WISC) using 12 years old subjects.

Bieri and Messerley (1957) obtained significant relations between Embedded figures Test (EFT) and extroversive-introversive Rorschach scores.

Goodenough and Karp (1961) studied to test the hypotheses that some intellectual and perceptual tests have a common requirement for overcoming embedding contexts, and that relationships obtained between measures of field-dependence and standard tests of intelligence are based on this common factor. A number of cognitive tests, including the WISC and standard tests of field dependence, were administered to eighty children (age 9 to 12 years) of a Public School in Brooklyn, New York. Two factor analyses were conducted on matrices of correlations between cognitive tests. The results tend to support both hypotheses.

Crutchfield, Woodworth and Alberchta (1958), Messick and Damarin (1964) found that field dependent individuals were displayed a better memory for faces.

Vaught's (1965) study was concerned with investigating the relationship of role identification and ego-strength to sex differences in Rod-and-Frame performance. A total of 180 subjects (90 male and 90 female) from Saint Louis University, were given the RFT (Witkin, et al., 1962) after having been asigned to one of 18 identity groups on the basis of their relative position on both the ego-strength scale and the femininity scale. All predictions were confirmed by the results. It was concluded that within the general population males were more field independent than females. However, it was argued that since role identification as well as ego-strength influences an individual to perceive the environment in a field-independent manner, these differences between males and females are best conceptualized as reflecting variations in role identification and ego-strength.

Pedersen (1965) scored a Sentence Completion Test for achievement motivation and for desire for security. The former measure correlated significantly with Rod-and-Frame Test, but the latter did not as expected, correlated negatively.

Kato (1965) applied the Rod-and-Frame Test to male Japanese students and obtained correlation of 0.4 to 0.5 with several social adjustment scores on he Guilford Personality Inventory; the figures for women were lower.

Pedersen was Wender (1968) conducted a study of field dependence and personality. Thirty boys were rated at nursery school, between 2 and 6 years, for various behaviour clusters including: seeking and accepting physical contact, seeking attention and help, orality, and sustained autonomous and directed play. At 6+ they were given Children's Embedded Figures Test, WISC and Kagan's Categorization Test. Rather small and irregular correlations, but in the expected direction, were obtained between all four clusters and CEFT, WISC performance (not verbal), and with Kagan's relational (non analytic) score.

Gardner and Moriarty (1968) working with 9-13 year olds, found few significant correlations between Embedded figures Test or Children's Embedded Figures Test and Rorschach or Holtzman blots or Clinical Ratings. They attempted to explain this, post hoc, as due to the complexity to personality organization in adolescence.

Adeval, Silverman and McGough (1968) obtained no significant relations between Rod-and-Frame Test and Minnesota Multiphasic

Personality Inventory, Barron's Ego-strength or Taylor's Anxiety Scale, apart from slight tendency for field dependents to score higher on the MMPI scale.

Vernon (1972) studied the distinctiveness of field independence. The subjects were large groups of boys and girls at Grade 8 level from Junior High Schools in Calgary, Alberta. Eight spatial or field independence measure together with reference tests of abilities and achievements, interest, and personality qualities were administered and showed that group paper-and pencil tests do not define a factor distinct from general intelligence (g) the spatial ability or visualization (s) when intelligence is held constant, such test show significant residual correlations with interests, though few test with personalty. However the Rod-and-Frame Test may involve a distinctive visuokinesthetic factor, since it gives a different pattern of correlations with other variables, which differs also in the two sexes.

Bowd (1975) studied the relationship between perceptual egocentrism and field dependence in early childhood. Fifty three kindergarten children were administered tests of inductive reasoning and field dependence and a series of perceptual egocentrism tasks. The principal expectation of the study, that field dependence would relate positively to perceptual egocentrism, was confirmed.

Goodenough's (1976) review of the literature relating individual differences in field dependence to learning and memory suggests the following conclusions: (a) field dependent subjects are dominated by the salient cues in concept attainment problems, whereas field independent subjects sample more fully from the available cue set; (b) field dependent subjects tend to use "spectator" approaches to learning, whereas field independent subjects more often use "participant" approaches; (c) field independence is related to frequency of dream recall; (d) field dependence is related to the magnitude of stress effects on learning and memory; (e) field independence is related to performance, effectiveness under conditions of intrinsic motivation; (f) field dependence is related to the effectiveness of negative reinforcement; and (g) incidental learning of social information is greater among field dependent than among field independent subjects.

In a recent review, Davis and Frank (1979) concluded that field independent and field dependent individuals differ not only in the cognitive processes they use, but also in the effectiveness of their performance. Specifically, they summarized past research which indicates that a field dependent learners display less efficient memory than field independent learners. One possible explanation of the poorer memory performance of field dependent individuals, as compared to field independent individual, is that field dependent learners process information rigidly, which results in the inefficient use of cues to trigger recall of past information.

Vectoria (1980) conducted a study on Verbal instruction and personality factors in perceptual performance. Personality types (introversion, extroversion) as determined by the Eysenck Personality Inventory and cognitive style. Experiments were carried out on a selected group of 66 technical students including introvert and extrovert and analytic and synthetic subjects who were subjected to a set of hidden figures and reversible images. Data show that the short duration sets created by barbel instructions and pre-training interacted with nature of task and other long term individual characteristics such as individual strategy, cognitive style and introversion and extroversion features.

Panek (1982) investigated the relationship between field dependence/independence and personality in older adults, the Group Embedded Figures Test and the Hand test were administered to 64 community-living, female, older adults raging from 60 to 81 years. Seven low but significant correlations were obtained between personality variables and the field dependence/independence dimension, In general, findings were both consistent and inconsistent with the theoretical assumptions with personality/behavioral characteristics that the field dependence/independence construct which suggests the personality relationships appear to change with old age.

Flexer and Roberge (1983) conducted a longitudinal investigation of field dependence/independence and the development of formal operational thought. The Group Embedded Figures Test and Paper and Pencil Measures of three formal operations schemes were administered to 120 pupils three times at one-year intervals. Analyses of correct responses indicated that the impact of field dependence/independence on the development of formal operational thought, apart from that explained by IQ differences was inconsequential.

Goodenough, Oltman and Cox (1987) conducted a study on nature of individual difference in field-dependence. The subjects were

199 females between the ages of 18 and 50. It was found that individual differences in field dependence were related to the Embedded Figures Test as expected but they were just as highly related to many other tests of Spatial-Visual Abilities. These relationships appeared due to the constancy component of he Rod-and-Frame Test.

Indian Studies

Bhatnagar and Rastogi (1985) conducted a study on cognitive style and basic-ideal disparity. The Self-concept Scale developed by Rastogi (1978) and the Embedded Figures Test developed by Witkin (1950) were administered to 192 Science Post-graduates of Lucknow University, India. Results indicate that the self is most significantly linked with cognitive style.

Studies on Personality and Reflection/Impulsivity Cognitive Style

Western Studies

The impulsive individual has been characterized as retaliative, risk-taking and emotionally uncontrolled (Kagan, 1965; Kagan and Kogan, 1970) in contrast to the reflective person who attempts to solve problems in a deliberate fashion; considers alternative solutions or choices and manifests greater impulse control (Kagan and Kogan, 1970; Messer, 1970).

Drew, Colquhoun and Long's (1958) study indicated that introverts, like Kagan's reflective children, perform tasks slowly and accurately whereas extroverts tend to be quick and inaccurate (impulsive).

Research don by Kagan (1965) on behavioural observations on 36 impulsive and reflective children in Fels Experimental Nursery School, Showed that the reflective child showed higher standards of intellectual tasks and could focus on an activity for a longer time. This may be due to the child's ability to perceive more or due to the ability to recall more than the impulsive child. The reflective children seemed to have a strong tendency to avoid peer group interaction and to be initially afraid in an unfamiliar social interaction. The impulsive child responds quickly and thus may make more errors in learning situations in recall tasks on inability to organize which may affect the total performance.

Kagan (1965) found that reflective children have performed better than impulsive children on reading tasks.

Kagan (1966) found that the reflective child is a low risk child who avoids situations that are potentially dangerous. The reflective child on the whole gave more correct responses, persisted longer on a task than his impulsive counterpart. The impulsive child on the other hand tended to be less tense and more casual in his responses and in a hurry to complete the task.

Kagan and Kogan (1970) reported that the sociability and active, motoric behavior of the impulsive child, the solitary achievement orientation of the reflective child suggest that perhaps these children might be more broadly differentiated as extroverts and introverts.

Messer (1970) studied the effect of anxiety over intellectual performance on reflection/impulsivity in children. Anxiety was aroused experimentally by having children fail in an intellectual task, and it's effects on decision time and errors on a match-to-sample task were assessed. The inducted anxiety resulted in longer decision gives for both impulsive and reflective children and in fewer errors for the impulsive who increased in response time. This finding supported the proposition that anxiety over intellectual performance is one antecedent of a reflective cognitive disposition.

Thomas (1971) found that among 7 year-old boys impulsive displayed more aggression than reflectives on a modification of Buss's Aggression Machine which employed noise as the noxious stimulus.

Lewise, Rausch, Goldberg and Dodd (1988), Ward (1968), Eska and Black (1971) found that IQs and errors on Matching Familiar Figures (MFF) are negatively and significantly related, the relationship established between IQs and latencies is inconsistent.

Siegal, Kirasic and Kilburg (1973) found that reflectives revealed superior short-term visual memory on a visual recognition task in which the child had to recall which of two similar pictures had been presented previously.

Kopfstein (1973) studied risk-taking behaviour and cognitive style. From a group of 60 fourth-grade children, 40 were classified as either reflective or impulsive based on Kagan's Matching Familiar Figures Task. These children then participated in a risk-taking situation. It was predicted that impulsive children would take more risks than reflective ones. Only a small, non-significant relationship was found between cognitive style and risk-taking behaviour, with impulsive tending to take more risks on one measure and fewer on another.

Schleifer and Douglas (1973) found that young children characterized as immature in their moral judgements were also impulsive while reflective subjects evidenced more mature moral judgement. Similarly, Caring (1970) reported a significant relationship between cognitive style and moral judgement in fifth graders and speculated that IQ may have accounted for this observation.

Kagan (1965) and Finch, Peszzuti, Montgomery, and Kemp (1974) found there was no relationship between intelligence and reflection/impulsivity.

Block, et al (1974) found Matching Familiar Figures classification to relate to q-sort items such as vital, energetic, lively, inhibited and constricted, physically cautious, rapid personal tempo and aggressive physically or verbally. These items imply the construct of extroversion-introversion.

Weiner and Berzonsky (1975) assessed selective attention in second, fourth, and sixth-grade reflective and impulsive children (Central New York School) with an incidental learning task. By the sixth grade, reflective children displayed less incidental learning and greater central learning than impulsive children. Reflective children showed a trade-off incidental learning for central learning but impulsive children did not appear to attend selectively. The findings were related to Hagen's 2-stage model of selective attention.

Cairns and Harbison (1975) conducted a study on impassivity: self report and performance measure. A sample of 98 boys, age 11-12 years, completed the Junior Eysenck Personality Inventory (JEPI) and were individually adminstered Kagan's Matching Familiar Figures Test of reflection/impulsivity. Four groups were formed on the basis of median splits on two indices of impulsivity and a two-way analysis of variance was carried out against Eysenck's personality dimensions and an additional impulsivity factor derived from the same inventory. The fact that no main effects or interactions were obtained for any self-report measure.

Brodzinsky's (1975) study showed that young impulsive boys smiled and laughed more to humorous materials which depicted aggressive behavior than did reflective boys. This may be suggestive of impulsive greater emotional stability - also an indicator of the less socialized child-or their particular responsivity to, and lesser need to control against, the impact of aggressive stimuli.

Bannigan and Ash (1977) research indicater that reflective children perform significantly better o the Wechsler Intelligent Scale for children than impulsive ones. New paral Messer and Broadzinsky (1979) studied the relationship of conceptual tempo to fantasy and overt aggression and it's control, in order to test the generalizability of this cognitive style to domains of social and pesonality functioning. Fifth grade boys and girls (n=127) from Central New Jersey, were administered and Matching Familiar Figures Test and Projective Measure of Factasy Aggression and it's control and were rated socio-metrically by peers and teachers on physical, verbal, and indirect forms of overt aggression. While reflective and impulsive children did not differ in degree of factasy aggression expressed, impulsive children especially boys, were found to exercise less control over their aggres-sive thoughts than the other 3 conceptual tempo groups. Impulsive and slow-inaccurate children were also more overtly aggressive, especially in comparison with fast accurates. In addition, fantasy aggression predicted overt aggression in impulsive but bot in reflectives.

Adejumo (1979) studied conceptual tempo and visual perceptual ability of some Nigerian children. Two hundred male children (7 and 9 year) from four Public Schools in Oshogbo, Oyo State, Nigeria were classified into four groups (Impulsive, Reflective, Fast-accurate, Slow-inaccurate) based on performance on modified Matching Familiar Figures Test. Subjects were also tested on object-comparison and visual-recognition tasks. Performance on modified matching familiar figures correlated significantly with performance on visual perceptual task. Seven year old subjects in the reflective and fast-accurate groups were superior in performance on the visual perceptual tasks.

Finch and Kendall (1979) examined the relationship between cognitive impulsivity assessed by Kagan's Matching Familiar Figures Test and impulsive behaviour, but the findings are mixed. Cognitively "impulsive" boys were rated as less considerate and less task-oriented than "reflective" boys and "impulsive" girls were rated more distract-ible than "reflective" girls.

Larsen (1980) studied cognitive tempo and intellectual performance in college students. Twenty four subjects were given the adult version of Kagan's Matching Familiar Figures Test and Advanced Progressive Matrices (1962) Set II. Neither errors nor latencies on the Matching Familiar Figures Test were significantly correlated with scores on the Advanced Progressive Matrices. These data suggest that the relationship between intellectual performance and scores on the Matching Familiar Figures Test for college students is different than that of the relationship for children.

Wiedl and Bathge (1981) reported that cognitive impulsive children's dysfunctional aspects of performance on intelligence tasks were analyzed for their compensativity with the Raven's Coloured Progressive Matrices. Subjects were classified for their impulsivity/ reflectivity with a median split of the Matching Familiar Figures Test optimizing testing conditions included differential feedback procedures or specific instructions to verbalise IQ and measures of frequency and duration of looking behaviour were the dependent measures. Result yield only a non-significant compensatory tendency for IQ.

Lajoie and Shore (1987) determined whether 52 high - IQ 10 the grade students (mean IQ 120) could be described as slow and accurate/ inaccurate or fast and accurate/inaccurate with regard to intellectual performance, using the Matching Familiar Figures Test. No significant differences in mean IQ were found among the groups.

Indian Studies

Agarwal and Srivastava (1981) studied the significance of time perspective in reflection/impulsivity. Sixty six college students were adminstered an Indian version of Matching Familiar Figures Test and a Story Writing Test that measured temporal orientation. It was found that 4 groups of subjects, exhibiting reflective, impulsive, fast accurate and slow inaccurate conceptual style differed significantly in their future orientation scores. Specifically, reflective subjects were significantly more future oriented whereas impulsive were significantly more present time oriented.

Achhpal and Mistry (1981) assessed the cognitive styles of 50 pre schoolers using the Kansas Reflection impulsivity Scale for Pre Schoolers. Teachers assessed their children on their ability to organize, observe and classify, understand auditory and language oriented factors. Results showed that impulsive subjects were below their age level expectancy in terms of learning abilities. Subjects classified as reflective were either above or at their age level expectancy. Reflective expectancy was shy, has few friends and did not participate in group activities.

Studies on Locus of Control and Creativity

Western Studies

Since its introduction (Phares, 1957), the concept of internal-external control has proved to be a highly useful personality dimension for understanding the role of reinforcement in a wide variety of behaviour situations.

Rotter and Mulry (1965) found a positive relation between internality and preference to perform in skill rather than in chance situations.

James (1965) found that internals were more persistent at a complex logical puzzle.

Davis and Phares (1967) found that internals more actively seek information relevant to problem-solving.

Brecher and Denmark (1969) reported that females who scored internal were more fluent than external females.

Ducette and Wolk (1972) found that externals tend to exhibit less persistence at tasks.

Gavurin and Murgatroyd (1973) found that internal females, but not males, performed better than external females on a single - solution anagram problem-solving task.

Bolen and Torrance (1978) noted that external subjects were more fluent than either internal subject or mixed locus of control and were significantly more creative over-all.

Richmond and Serna (1980) studied creativity and locus of control among Mexican College students. Torrance Test of Creativity and the Rotter I-E Scale was used to measure creativity and locus of control. Results indicated that external students were more creative.

Indian Studies

Agarwal and Verma (1977) found that highly creative students believe that rewards are contingent upon one's efforts and are not governed by chance, luck, fate or systems.

Studies on Locus of Control and Field Dependence/Independence Cognitive Styles

Western Studies

Crandall and Lacey (1972) found that internal-external perceptions were related to three performance measures on the Witkin's Embedded Figures Test in a sample of 50 elementary school age children. When the effects of age and IQ were partialled out of the internality-embedded figures relationships, prediction was reduced or males but remained at significant levels for females. Although internal females committed as many error as external females, they were able to identity more figures correctly and in less time than their external peers.

Davis (1982) found that internal control is directly related to field independence while external control is related to field dependence.

Marx, Howard and Winne (1987) conducted a study to explore relations of field dependence/independence and locus of control with student's perceptions of a teachers' use of instructional cues and the cognitive responses the teacher intends students to make to these cues. Another purpose was to examine how cognitive style and student's ability to perceive instructional cues and cognitive responses jointly relate to students's achievement. Data from 87 students in Grade 6 indicated that the two cognitive style measures relate neither to students/s perception of instructional cues not to cognitive responses. However, measures of both perceptions were related to achievement, even after statistically controlling for verbal ability. Results are interpreted in terms of student's perceptions as mediating links between teaching events and student's achievement of curricular objectives.

Indian Studies

Tripathi and Tripathi (1984) examined perceptual dependence in relation to approval motive, socio economic status (SES) and locus of control. The sample for the study consisted of undergraduate students of Gorakhpur University. A low and high approval X low and high SESX internal and external control (2^3) factorial design was used. 10 subjects were randomly assigned to each treatment condition and tested on Oltman's portable Rod-and-Frame Test (PRFT). Results showed that all the main effects (approval, SES, and Locus of control) were significant. The interaction between approval X SES, approval X locus of control, and approval X SES X locus of control was found significant. Approval motive, socio-economic status and locus of control jointly influenced perceptual dependence.

Studies on Locus of Control and Reflection/impulsivity Cognitive Style

Western Studies

Shipe (1971) found a significant but moderate correlation between reflectivity and internal locus of control in a sample of vocational school boys but not in a similar sample of institutionalized boys.

Campbell and Douglas (1972) observed that reflective boys were more likely than impulsive to tell stories on a projective test that involved expectation of success in meeting of threat of frustration. By contrast, the impulsive subjects passively accepted the inevitability of such events.

Messer (1972) found that the superior performance in academic-intellectual tasks of children with an internal locus of control may be due to greater reflectivity on the part of internals.

Berzonsky (1974) found no difference in locus of control between reflectives and impulsives in first and second graders.

Massari (1975) reported only a trend toward internality among reflective first and third grade black children.

INFLUENCE OF ENVIRONMENTAL FACTORS ON CREATIVITY AND COGNITIVE STYLES

Studies on Home Environment and Creativity

Western Studies

According to Getzels and Jackson (1961) parents and the home atmosphere appear to be more instrumental in fostering or hindering the creative talents of their children than more other determinants. Saran (1970) also concluded that individual development of child with regard to curiosity, creativity, constructiveness and practical competence depends largely upon the presence of proper environment at home.

Several studies have been performed to investigate the relationship of va..ious factors in home environment to general creativity. Baldwin (1949) found that parental democracy stimulates creativity and imaginativeness among children.

Teran (1954) in his comparison of creativity as opposed to non-creative gifted children showed that the non-creative came from homes having more stress, more conflict, and less interest in achievement than homes of creative subjects.

Watson (1957) compared the personalities of 44 children, 6 to 11 years of age, from homes rated as "loving" but with strict parental discipline, and 34 children of the same age from homes rated as having an "extraordinary degree of permissiveness. On the basis of projective tests and teachers' ratings, the children from the more permissive families were rated as having significantly greater spontaneity, originality, and creativity, accompanied by more initiative and independence, better socialization, friendliness to others, and less inner hostility. All the children in this study had an IQ of 110 or above, as determined by a vocabulary test.

Roe (1960) found parents of the social scientists to be over protective, firm, and control, even if not overt, was very evident.

Orienstein (1961) reported no evidence about the positive relationship between the permissive child-rearing attitudes of mothers and highly creativity after the child's IQ and the mother's need for socially approved behaviour were partialed out.

Weisberg and Springer (1961) reported a correlation of 0.5 between the integrity of the father - child relationship and the level of creative test performance. Compulsivity in the mother as rated by psychiatric interviews was found to be negatively correlated with creativity test scores in children.

In Singer's (1961) study, members of the high fantasy group had significantly more contact with their parents and also chosen one parent (usually the father) than did those of the low fantasy group, who stated that they liked both parents equally.

Getzels and Jackson (1962) found that mothers of high creative children less often than mothers of high IQ children report worries about the dangers in the world, recollections of insecurity in their own childhood, admiration for conventional qualities in children, vigilance regarding their children's school performance and restrictions on their children's independence.

Mackinnon (1962) examining the life history of creative individuals observed that not all of them had happy homes and favourable life circumstances and some underwent brutal treatment at the hands of sadistic fathers.

Stein (1963) reported some interesting results based on the study of biographics of chemists who were engaged in industrial research. His more creative subjects said that they were more distant from either parent and from adults in general than do his less creative subjects. Parents of more creative subjects were more inconsistent in their attitudes towards them than those of less creative subjects.

Nichols (1964) reported that mothers who were rated high on authoritarian child rearing attitudes tended to have children who were low in creativity and originality.

Drevdahl (1964) testing psychologists, and Mackinnon (1964) testing architects found that their more creative subjects were given more independence and responsibility during childhood than the average child.

Barbe (1964) studied the personal adjustment, family background, and school achievement of 65 highly gifted children and 65 moderately gifted children. The sample drawn from throughout the State of Ohio included 31 matched pairs of boys and 34 matched pair of girls. The highly creative subjects were found in the more affluent and the more highly educated families.

In their assessment of the home environment of highly creative adolescents, Holland (1961), Getzels and Jankson (1961) and Nichols (1964) noted that the parents were less authoritarian and stressed openness to experience and an enthusiasm for life, in contrast to the parents of the highly intellectual youths who promoted good or conforming behaviour and studiousness in their children.

After interviewing and testing 48 ten-year-old boys and their mothers, Dyk and Witkin (1965) found a significantly, negative relationship between the child's degree of differentiation and the degree to which the mother stressed conformity and limited her son's curiosity.

Talented architects in Mackinnon's study (1965) reported having as children an unusual amount of freedom in making decisions and exploring their environment; they experienced neither over protection nor rejection from their parents, but at the same time parents set definite standards of conduct and values and provided a model for identification.

Dryer and Wells (1966) concluded that the parents of the more creative children (as assessed by TTCT (showed less consensus in family values, and more role tensions than the parents of low creatives. However, the extent to which the parents granted autonomy to the child did not differentiate the two group of parents.

Nuttal's (1969) study reports the relationship between creativity and parental acceptance and autonomy. Mehdi's Test of Creativity Thinking (MTCT) and teachers ratings were used to measure creativity of 180 sixth grade boys, and categorized them as high and low creative boys. The parents of these boys answered the Parental Attitude Research Instrument (PARI) and the Maryland Parent Attitude Survey (MPAS). The high and low creative boys also answered the Child's Report of Parental Behaviour Inventory (CRPBI). It was found that (1) high creativity would be positively correlated with high parental acceptance and autonomy, when teacher's ratings and the CRPBI were used but when the MTCT were used, it was not found; (2) teachers' rating of creativity were positively correlated with the maternal firm control factor of the CRPBI; (3) the correlation between the total MTCT scores and teacher's ratings of creativity was not significant.

Silverberg (1970) designed a study to investigate relationships between children's perception of certain basic parental child-rearing behaviour or attitudes namely acceptance and permissiveness and the creativity of these children "Torrance Tests of Creativity Thinking" and the "Cornell Parent Behaviour Description" were used as a measure of creativity and of children's perceptions of parental behaviour. The subjects of the study were 205 middle class IV grade boys and girls selected from 6 Pubic Elementary Schools in New York city. Subjects in the superior range of intelligence were chosen. Analysis of data revealed (1) a significant relationship between father acceptance and fluency for boy; (2) girls' perception of their mothers as more accepting than boys; (3) rejection of hypotheses predicting positive relationship between the extent to which children perceived their mothers and fathers as accepting and permissive and the creativity of these children; (4) progressive decrease in father's acceptance with increase from the lowest to the higher levels of fluency; and (5) at the highest levels of fluency, fluency was associated with the high levels of acceptance.

Eisenman and Foxman (1970) examined to know the family patterns associated with creativity. Subjects were 75 undergraduates from Temple University. They were asked to provide a large amount of information about their family on a questionnaire. Three creativity measures were presented in the following order: brick use, pencil use, and polygon preference. Results report that students having spent most of their lives with both parents would be more creative than spending most their life with one or none and living at home while attending college would be negatively associated with creativity.

Wade (1971) found that parents of creative adolescents tend to be better educated and more interested and supportive to their children.

Walberg (1971) obtained data from 3000 adolescents on self-reported creativity, biographical variables and IQ. He found that adolescent creativity is associated with stimulating home environment.

Heilbein (1971) found that adolescents with highly controlling and low nurturant mothers lack in creativity than those with mothers rated as converse.

Swan and Stavros (1973) studied child rearing practices associated on the development of the cognitive skills of children in low socio-economic areas. Parents were evaluated in relations to 4 dimensions; parental philosophy and values, perception of the child feelings of competence and verbal interaction. In these families a helpful and encouraging attitude was maintained by parents. Children were perceived as curious adventurous, creative, and independent learners.

Dewing (1973) studied some characteristics of the parents of creative twelve-year-olds. A battery of creativity tests was given to 394 seventh grade children in Perth, Western Australia. Information obtained from parents indicated that those with highly creative children preferred a complex and stimulating environment for themselves and for their children. The educational level of the mother and unusual religious beliefs were related to creativity test scores. The were more working mothers in the creative group than in the control group matched for IQ, sex, and school. Mothers of creative children held more equalitarian child rearing attitudes and permitted their children more contact with influences outside the home. The characteristics of the parents were more closely related to the creativity of the like-sex children, and this relationship was stronger with respect to the children's creative performance than to their scores on the creativity tests.

Aldous (1975) reports association of girls' novel solutions to controlling behaviour from fathers. Maternal controlling behaviours, however, were generally associated with less original solution among both girls and boys. Fathers in their demands seemed to be setting standards for more originality while maternal assistance had the effect of narrowing the children's freedom to be original.

Moore and Bulbutian (1976) found that subjects in the presence of an aloof, critical adult were less likely to display incidental task related to curiosity and exploratory behaviour and were less inclined to venture guesses as to the identity of objects than subjects in the presence of friendly and supportive adult.

Shmukler (1982-83) conducted a follow-up study of 73 third graders from an original sample of 114 mother-child pairs who were observed when the subjects were pre schoolers. It was concluded that an optimal balance between involvement, caring and warmth on the part of the part of the pre schooler's mother and a willingness to let the child explore at his/her own pace leads to future creative and imaginative expression.

Fu, Moran, Sawyers and Milgram (1983) examined the relationship between pre schooler's creativity and parental child rearing attitudes. Their results fail to indicate any significant relationship between creativity in children and specific parental variables, as measured through the Parent Attitude Research Instrument.

Write (1987) presented a ecological model of the interaction of home and school environments in the development of creative thinking skills in young children. The model emphasizes reciprocal interactions between children's physical and social environments and the primary influence of the family on their developing creativity.

Indian Studies

Sinha and Sharma (1978) obtained significant negative correlations between creativity index and home, health and emotional adjustment, signifying that the high creatives were better adjusted in those fields. They further observed that the high and the low creatives could be significantly differentiated in home and health adjustment scores.

A study is designed by Asha (1983) to see the effect of maternal employment on the creativity of children. The sample consists of 510 boys and 590 girls (mean age 14.66 and 14.43 years respectively) from 18 Secondary Schools in Trivandrum Educational district. Wallach and Kogan Tests of Creativity Thinking Abilities and a Personal Data Blank were given to the selected sample. The analysis of the data shows that maternal employment is a factor that facilitates development of creativity in children.

Cross Cultural Studies

Anderson and Anderson (1965), in a cross cultural study of creativity among elementary and Junior high schools children, have found that creative expression is more frequent in cultures characterized by less authoritarian attitudes toward child rearing and social relationships.

Straus and Straus (1968) theorized that children's creativity varies according to the degree to which the child's family role requires conformity to conventional norms. Creativity was measured by the ability to generate ideas which might solve a puzzle presented to family groups. Data for 128 Indian and American Families showed that Indian children had lower scores than Americans. Girls' scores were lower than boys in both societies. Sex differences in creativity were greatest in India. The Smaller sex difference in American sample was interpreted as reflecting the greatest freedom permitted to American girls. It was concluded that individual creativity is likely to increase as societies move toward a less restrictive normative code.

Studies on Home Environment and Field Dependence/Independence Cognitive Style

Although cognitive styles as a topic of psychological enquiry has had great popularity in the last two decades, relatively little systematic research has been carried out on the effect of parental and home background variables.

Western Studies

Dyk and Witkin (1965) found that positive influence on child's field independence of parent's emphasis on independence, self-reliance, and achievement.

Barclay, and Cusumano (1967) and Goldstein and Peck (1973) found children with father absent to be more field dependence than those with fathers present.

Witkin and Berry's (1975) study claim that the mothers imparting standards for internalization and regulation of impulses favour development of a child's field independence.

Kagan and Lawrence (1982) tested the relation of maternal reinforcement variables to children's reading and math achievement and field independence among 39 semi-rural low income Anglo-American mothers and their 7 to 9 years old children. Maternal reward punishment, and contingency generalized significantly across two novel behavioural tasks, and were more related to children's verbal than quantitative abilities. For all children, reading ability was associated with a rewarding, non-punitive, non-contingent mother. Math ability was not related to maternal award, but was related to a non-punitive non-contingent mother for boys.

Indian Studies

Paul (1986) conducted a study of cognitive styles in relation to age, achievement, home environment and social class. The sample consisted of 600 high school students of Home Science drawn from 9 schools of Agra city. Tests of Cognitive Preferences Styles. Achievement Test of Home Science, Social Class Scale an Home Environment Inventory were administered to subjects. The findings were as follows: 1) when the individuals do not differ on modes of preferences across the age, their cognitive styles will also remain immutable during the whole period and adolescence 2) the girls in general express preference for questioning mode of cognitive functioning in higher mental functions and mode of low achievement. 3) all the modes of cognitive preference were positively lively correlated, on levelling, the sequence of different modes of preference was "Questioning, Recall, Application and Principle." 4) the high achievers tend to impress high loadings on "Q-R" mode, while the low achievers on "R-Q" mode. 5) each of four modes of cognitive styles was positively and significantly correlated with home environment score.

Over View

The first section of review of related literature deals with contributions to the measurement of creativity and cognitive styles. It is apparent that measurement of children's creativity has attracted the attention of many Indian researchers and constructed some of the tests on the basis of well known Western contributors. In the case of cognitive styles, there exists a dearth of researchers in India, who contributed to the measurement of cognitive styles.

This information helps to know about the western and Indian researchers who have contributed to the measurement of creativity and cognitive styles. These literature help us understand the implications of constructing a test or scale and to know the utility of such instruments in the present context.

The second section presented the studies on inter-relation between creativity and cognitive styles. Very few Indian studies on inter-relation between creativity and field dependence/independence cognitive style were reported and no Indian studies were available with regard to reflection/impulsivity cognitive style. So, the present enquiry attempts to see the relationship between creativity and cognitive styles in tribal and non-tribal children.

The studies on influence of demographic factors (ethnicity, age and sex) on creativity and cognitive styles were presented in the third section. Under ethnicity, the Western and Indian studies relating to social class, race, socio cultural disadvantage, tribal and non-tribal groups, rural and urban groups were presented. Apart from these the cross-cultural research was also reported with regard to creativity and cognitive styles.

On the whole, the research studies on ethnicity and creativity and cognitive style are not many, particularly with reflection/impulsivity cognitive style.

There are very few studies related to age and creativity in Western and Indian culture, with regard to sex difference and creativity, the findings of Western and Indian studies are varied and not conclusive.

Only a few Western studies were presented on age and sex differences and cognitive styles but no Indian studies were available on this aspect. So, the present study is directed towards certain demographic factors like ethnicity, age and sex influencing creativity and cognitive styles in tribal and non-tribal children.

The fourth section reported on influence of psychological factors (personality and locus of control) on creativity and cognitive styles. Considerable research in Western countries and India was reported to identify the personality characteristics of different types of creative persons. But, the generated research data is equivocal and inconsistent. Research with regard to pesonality and field dependence/independence and reflection/impulsivity in India is still inadequate and infancy in growth.

Very few Western and Indian studies were conducted on locus on control and creativity and cognitive styles. The present study is therefore focused upon certain psychological factors mainly personality and locus of control influencing creativity and cognitive styles in tribal and non-tribal children. It is expected that this research data will be helpful in throwing some light on this issue.

The review of literature presented in the fifth section is on the influence of environmental factors (home environment) on creativity and cognitive styles. Some studies were carried out in Western countries on home environment and creativity. But, very few systematic Indian research and cross-cultural studies were conducted on this aspect. Results of different studies are not conclusive.

Studies conducted in Western and Indian cultures on field dependence/independence and home environment are very scanty. No significant study was made on reflection/impulsivity and home environment in Western and Indian countries. The present study therefore warranted as it emphasizes the environment factor (home environment) influencing creativity and cognitive styles in tribal and non-tribal children.

On the whole, research on the relationship of creativity and cognitive styles and with different factor has brought out inconsistent and inconclusive results which necessitate further research. Consistent and appropriate findings are necessary to enlighten the teachers, parents, administrators and all concerned to work for the development of the creative potential and cognitive styles of the child to the fullest extent possible. The present study is aimed at finding out the effect of certain factors on creativity and cognitive styles in tribal and non-tribal children.

3

METHODOLOGY

GENERAL PLAN

The major objective of the research study is to determine the influence of certain demographic (ethnicity, age and sex), psychological (personality and locus of control) and environmental (home environment) factors on creativity and cognitive styles of tribal and non-tribal children.

In the first stage the tools to measure creativity (verbal and non-verbal), cognitive styles (field dependence/independence and reflection/impulsivity), personality, locus of control and home environment were selected and tested on a pilot sample of 30 subject (15 Sugali tribal and 15 non-tribal) to establish relevant psychometric properties.

The selected research tools are as follows:

1. Mehdi's (1973) Test of Verbal and Non-verbal Creative Thinking (adapted by the investigator).
2. Embedded Figures Test.
3. Matching Familiar Figures Test (developed by the Investigator).
4. Adapted version of Children's Personality Questionnaire (Siddamma, 1979) (modified by the Investigator).
5. Rotter's (1966) Internal and External control scale (adapted and modified by the investigator).

6. Adapted version of Home Environment Inventory (Manjuvani and Kalyani, 1987) (modified by the Investigator).

In the second stage, the tools were administered on a final sample of 200 student (100 non-tribal selected from 10, 11 and 12 years age group (5th, 6th and 7th standards) in schools of Chittoor district, Andhra Pradesh.

The data generated on the sample was subjected to qualitative and quantitative statistical analysis. Qualitative analysis consists of evaluation of descriptive statistics for all the variables. Quantitative analysis consists of Step-wise Multiple Regression Analysis in order to understand the regression of the independent variables on the dependent variables. In this, the independent variables used are age, sex, locus of control and home environment. The dependent variables are creativity and cognitive styles. A Multiple Regression Analysis was planned to establish the relative contribution of the independent variables to the variance in the dependent variables. The quantitative analysis also includes the application of the Chi-square, t-test, f-test Correlation Coefficients, Discriminant Function Analysis. Apart from these Personality Profiles were also drawn.

In this chapter, the details of the methods followed in the study namely, ethnographic profile of Sugali tripe, construction of research tools, sample for final study, data collection, scoring of the instruments and various statistical techniques employed in the analysis of data are presented.

To know the characteristic features of Sugali tribals, the ethnographic profile is given as follows:

ETHNOGRAPHIC, PROFILE ON SUGALI TRIBE OF CHITTOOR DISTRICT, ANDHRA PRADESH

In Andhra Pradesh State there are 33 notified scheduled tribes spread all over (Census of India, 1981). The population of tribals in Andhra Pradesh, according to 1981 Census, is about 31,76,001 (16,18,689 males and 15,57,312 females) i.e. 6.15 per cent of the total population of India. The tribes like Koya, Yanadi, Sugali, Yerukala, Gond and Konda, Doras have the largest population in Andhra Pradesh.

Note : Census of 1991 is not available. So the population figures are based on 1981 census.

Among the tribes living in the hilly and plain areas of Andhra Pradesh, the Sugalis comprise one of the numerically dominant tribes. They are predominantly found in Anantapur, Chittoor, Guntur, Mahboobnagar, Krishna, Kurnool, Warangal and Adilabad districts. According to 1981 Census, the Sugali population of Andhra Pradesh is 595, 632 males and 562, 710 females.

Sugalis are inhabiting the hilly and forest areas of Chittoor district in Rayalaseema region and particularly they are concentrated in the Western Talukas of Chittoor. According to the Census of 1981 in Chittoor, the Sugali population is 7,734 males and 7,456 females. The Sugalis are known by different names such as Banjaras, Lambani, Brinjari, Vanjari, Boyapani, Sugali or Sukali in different regions of India. Pratap (1968) is of opinion that Sugalis might have been a corruptive form of the Sanskrit word Sugwala (good cow-herd). But Ramachandra Reddy, M. (1984) reports that some Sugalis from Sugalimitta and other villages of Chittoor district feel that the word "Sugali" is derived from the word "Supari" meaning "Betelnut" (supari) since their ancestor once traded supari.

Origin

The origin and history and of Sugalis is not clear and have several meanings. Enthoven (1920) feels that these people have connections with other castes and tribes but Sugalis strictly opposed this idea of their mixed origin. It is known from the several earlier literature, that Sugalis of Lambadis or Banjaras are not the natives of South India. Thurston (1909) stated that the Sugali culture and language indicated that they hailed from Northern India. Their folklore depicts them to be the descendants of Rajput Stock.

Location

Sugalis generally stay in the hill or in the forest region in the inaccessible parts. During transitional phase, some of their houses are situated near the main road and hence, they are getting exposed to the civilized world.

Economy

Sugalis who were once nomadic are currently practising agriculture besides forest work and live in permanent dwellings. Some of them have become robberers during transition phase. Hence, they are often described as a criminal tribe. They also practise small scale business by selling salt, grain and other forest products including fruits, leaves, arrack etc. Forest economy includes the collection of forest products like tamarind, soapnit seeds (Shikakai), honey, hill brooms, firewood etc. They also prepare country liquor for their domestic use (to drink).

Occupation

Their chief occupation is selling of firewood, cultivation and cattle rearing. Some of them are agricultural labourers. They cultivate mainly groundnuts, cotton as well as other commercial crops. They also grow the cereals such as redgram, horsegram, blackgram and millets. Most of the Sugalis practise hunting of animals like rabbit and forest pig for the purpose of meat. At present some of the Sugalis are employees in Government institutions.

Income

Their annual income is below the poverty line*. Most of the people are found to have the annual income of Rs. 2,400 to Rs. 4,200.

Housing Conditions

Sugalis live in detached clusters of rude huts called "Thandas" located at some distance from villages, which are constructed mostly oblong, sometimes square thatched houses in rows with street in between. In some places unplanned pattern of houses without streets are also found. Thatched huts of Susalis consist of only one room with no way except the doorway. The same room is used for all purposes such as kitchen, dining, bed room, etc. Some Sugalis of economically well-off-have built improved houses with proper ventilation and more accommodation. In some of the areas Social Welfare department has constructed a systematic pattern of tiled houses for the Sugalis. For examples, they are at Sugalimitta, Ankisettipalli and Jandla.

Living Conditions

Sugalis are mostly living in primitive or barbarous conditions. There living conditions are very poor, without any adequate water, public latrines and other facilities for their living. They throw the waste

---

* Poverty line is annual household income of Rs. 6,400/- in rural areas and Rs. 7,300/- in the urban areas.

and rubbish in the pits locates outside the Thandas. Most of them do not have daily bath. Normally males takes bath once in two or three days whereas females once in a week. Males change their dress more frequently than females. When they suffer from fever and other aliments, generally they do not feel like going to hospitals or doctors, but they take indigenous medicines. Now-a-days the transitional Sugalis are improving their living conditions to some extent by various welfare measures.

Household Possessions

The families of the Sugalis use mostly earthernware and to some extent metalware as cooking utensils. They use mats, old clothes or bed sheets as bedding materials. Infants under two months are put in a bamboo cradle into which several old clothes are spread. After two months of age, children are put in usual hanging cradles made of old clothes or gunny bags. Almost every family owns a radio. A few of them have cycles and watches. Traditional type of dress, costumes, accessories and cosmetics are seen in some of the homes. A great majority of transitional Sugali families own more metal cooking vessels, possess cots, mattresses, pillows apart from the mats and bed sheets. Now they are giving importance to writing and reading materials like table, chair, news papers, pen/pencils, etc.

Racial Features

The Sugalis are strong and virile race with tall stature and fair complexion. Men are muscular and of medium height with Rajput features. They have light brown eyes and dark brown coloured hair with line texture.

Language and Literacy

Sugalis have their own dialect, which closely resembles the Marvari language of Rajasthan. But it lack script. In their language, some words of Dravidian language of surrounding regions are mixed. Probably these Sugalis, after coming to Andhra Pradesh due to cultural contact, also began speaking Telugu, Urdu, Kannada and other languages. Hence, they have become bilingual though basically illiterate. But, now-a-days, due to migration to sub-urban areas and the facilities provided by the Government they do represent some percentage among literates. Literacy rate is very low, but relatively it is slightly higher than the other tribal population. The level of literacy among Sugalis is mostly upto Secondary, excepting a few.

Groups

Sugalis constitute six important endogamous groups (Monograph series, Census of India, 1961) viz., Bhukya, Mude, Bhanavathi, Bavanath, Vaditya and Khorra who practise endogamous. Usually a Bhukya would not get a spouse from his own section/division. But, they are used to exchange between Bhukya and Mude. Bhukya and Bavanath, Bhukya and Vaditya, Bhukya and Khorra and Bhukya and Bhanavathi. But, in Chittoor district, it is observed that there are four sub-groups namely (1) Bhukya, (2) Mude, (3) Bhanavathi and (4) Khorra.

Names

Sugalis of Chittoor district and their names are very peculiar. The names are very similar and they add 'Nayak' after their names like Rama Nayak, Sundhar Nayak, Muniya Nayak, etc. The names of laides run as "Devi, Bhimli, Nanke"

Dress Pattern

The women wear a very peculiar skirt and coarse and red cotton cloth, embroidered in the border. Some small round mirror pieces are fixed all over the skirt. They wear blouses which are open at the back and are rich in embroidery work. They invariably cover their heads with another coloured piece of cloth. The men wear coloured or white handloom shirts and dhotis. They wear turban on their heads.

At present some change is observed in the dress pattern of women who are wearing sarees and blouses.

Ornaments

Females have numerous ornaments and include string of glass and beads, besides those of brass and other metals. The married women wear bangles of horns upto shoulders whereas unmarried upto elbow. They use different types of anklets and toe-rings. Some men wear only finger and toe-rings of silver.

The transitional Sugali women wear simple ornaments, like chain, bangles, ear and nose rings etc.

Food Habits

Their staple food is a coarse cake made of jowar or wheat. Some of them occasionally use rice. They are largely non-vegetarians. During festive occasions they prepare sweet with rice flour and jaggery. A few of them drink coffee or tea occasionally. They are fond of strong liquor. Both males and females chew pans.

Social Customs

Sugalis are very orthodox people. Their principal deity is Poleramma. They also worship Lord Venkateswara (Balaji). Offerings of money are made to this deity in anticipation of blessings. They sacrifice animals to Poleramma. They celebrate yearly functions like Jathara. The divided brothers meet once in a year in order to conduct the annual ceremony for the departed souls. They also assemble at various functions held at decided places. The expenditure for all these ceremonies is shared equally by all brothers. They also worship the dieters like Gangamma, Muthyalamma, Mariamma and so on. They sacrifice the goats, hens and other animals to all these deities in order to look after their Thandas from various evils such as epidemics and so on.

Law and Justice

Each Thanda has a headman called the "Nayak" whose word is the law and his office is hereditary. Each Thanda is under the control of a headman who is elected by the Thanda people. Whenever a problem arises or quarrels occurs, people go to him for seeking solution and they will abide by his judgement. He plays an important role and has all right to punish the guilty who involve in anti-social activities.

Marriage Practices

Marriage is universal in the Sugalis. Marriages are contracted within the same gotra or clan i.e. clan exogamy. Cross-cousin marriages are common and a few uncle-niece marriages are also observed. Monogamy is the rule but a few polygynous marriages are found due to barrenness of the first wife. Normally girls marry after attaining puberty and marriage age is early. In the case of males, they marry between 18 and 25 years. Marriage is done by negotiations. Sometimes love marriages are also practiced. Marriage by elopement is very rare. Widow remarriage is allowed. Divorce will be decided by their panchayat. Earlier marriage ceremony was for eight days but now they celebrate marriages within two days. Bride must pay some money and some articles to the girls's parents, called bride price. The bride price is different in different groups. It is Rs 450/- for Bhukia, Rs. 460/- for Mude and for Bhanavathi it is Rs. 450/- plus some articles. But, it was very less in the olden days.

Type of family

The basic kin unit of Sugalis is a nuclear family. Besides, there are extended & joint families. They are patrilocal, patrilineal and patriprotestal in authority. Generally the practice of polyandry is absent.

Child Rearing Practices

During pregnancy, the Sugalis practise pregnancy taboos relating to food and movement. A majority of the Sugalis desire to have 3 to 4 children. The preference for son as first child is very much intact in them. Generally, they perform religious ceremonies on children like purificatory ceremony after child's birth, ceremony associated with birth of a male child, cradling, name giving and tonsure ceremony. Prolonged breast feeding is a common practice and start to give supplementary foods at 7–12 months of age. Indigenous and magical treatment is very much prevalent when their children suffer from cold, cough, diarrhoea, scabies and measles etc. At present they are inclined towards allopathic treatment. A majority of the Sugali parents give less importance of personal cleanliness (cleaning teeth regularly, frequency of giving bath and changing clothes, etc.) of their children, when age of the child increases. Many Sugalis use scolding, spanking, deprivation of food and physical punishment as disciplinary measures to the children. At present some of the parents give emphasis to well education and employment to their children and wish them not to cultivate undesirable social habits.

CONSTRUCTION OF RESEARCH TOOLS

Mehdi's (1973) Test of Verbal And Non-Verbal Creative Thinking:

Recent advances in the area of creativity research have necessitated the development of suitable tools and devices to assess reliably the creative potential of pupils for their proper education and training. Mehdi (1973) has developed a test of creative thinking with verbal and non-verbal components and standardized it on Indian students. Hence, it is culture fair test. It was proposed to administer in the present investigation, with some adaptations.

The test battery is meant to identify creative talent at all stages of education, except pre-primary. The type of tasks included in the test were chosen so that they could be most easily and economically administered over a wide age range of sample starting from elementary school and going up of the graduate level.

The theoretical framework for the preparation of the test battery was provided by empirical studies on the nature of creativity. Especially useful in clarifying the concept of creativity has been the distinction. Guliford has made between two types of thinking. Guliford defines divergent thinking as a kind of mental operation in which we think in different directions, sometimes searching, sometimes seeking variety. Unlike convergent thinking, where information leads to one right answer or a recognised best or conventional answer, divergent production leads to novel responses to given stimuli. The unique feature of divergent thinking is that a variety of responses is produced. Guliford relates divergent thinking to certain well-known ability factors which seem to go with creative output. The primary traits related to divergent thinking and therefore, to creativity have been enumerated by Guliford as follows:

1. Sensitivity to problems, a trait best indicated by tests asking examinees to state defects or deficiencies in common implements, or in social institutions, or to state problems created by common objects or actions.
2. Fluency of thinking, which has to do with fertility of ideas.
3. Flexibility of thinking, consisting of two factors, namely, spontaneous flexibility defined as "the ability or disposition to produce a great variety of ideas, with freedom from inertia or from preservation," and adaptive flexibility which facilitates the production of a most unusual type of solution.
4. Originality, indicated by unusualness of responses, clever responses, or remote association and relationships. One must get away from the obvious, the ordinary, or conventional in order to make a good score.
5. Re-definition, a factor which causes an ability to give up old interpretation of familiar objects in order to use them or their parts in some new ways. Improvising, in general, probably reflects the ability of re-definition.
6. Elaboration, indicated by task in which the examinee is given one or two simple lines and told to construct on this foundation a more complex object.

In the preparation of the verbal and non-verbal tests of creativity, tasks pertaining to four of the six traits, viz., fluency, flexibility, originality and elaboration were used. The remaining two could not be included as the test would have become very time-consuming. Moreover, the four traits used in the test were considered to be the most important ones, and it was felt that taken together they would give a fairly valid information about the creative potential of the individual.

The test material consists of verbal and non-verbal tests of creative thinking booklets, manual and data scoring sheets.

Description of Verbal test of Creativity

The verbal Test of Creativity includes four activities namely, Consequences, Unusual Uses, New Relationships, and Product Improvement.

1. Consequences

It consists of three hypothetical situations. The subject is required to think as many consequences of these situations as he can, and write them under each situation in the space provided. The situations being hypothetical, minimize the effect of experience and also provide the subject with an unlimited opportunity to make responses. This activity encourages free play of imagination and originality.

2. Unusual Uses

It presents the subjects with the names of three common objects and requires him to write as many novel, interesting and unusual uses of these objects as he may think of. It measures the subject's ability to retrieve items of information from his personal information in storage. Evidently, it measures also the subject's ability to shift frames of reference to use the environment in an original manner.

3. New Relationships

It presents the subject with three pairs of words openly different, requires him to think and write as many novel relationships as possible between the two objects of each pair. It provides an opportunity for the free play of imagination and originality.

4. Product Improvement

In this activity the subject is asked to think of a simple model of particular animal and suggest addition of new things to it, to make it more interesting for the children to play.

An example is given on the test booklet for consequences, unusual uses and new relationships activities to acquaint the subject with the nature of task. Clear instructions and the time allowed for each activity are given in the test booklet itself.

Reported Psychometric Properties

Reliability

The test-retest reliabilities of the factor scores and also the total score were obtained on a rural and urban sample children (n=31). Both factor score and the total creativity score reliabilities are considerably high ranging from 0.896 to 0.959. These values are highly satisfactory. Inter-scorer reliability for the factor scores are found to range from 0.653 to 0.981.

Validity

The validity coefficients for factor scores and the total creativity score is high enough (significant at 0.01 level) to place confidence in the use of the test.

Description of Non-verbal Test of Creativity

The Non-verbal Test of Creativity is intended to measure the individual's ability to deal with figural content in a creative manner. Three types of activities are used for this purpose, viz.., Picture Construction, Incomplete Figures, and Triangles and Ellipses.

1. Picture Construction

This activity presents the subject with two simple geometrical figures, a semi-circle and rhomb, and requires him to construct an elaborate picture using each figure as an integral part. The subject is allowed to turn the page to use the figure in any way he likes for making the picture. Emphasis is put on originality and elaboration. Originality is emphasized by the instruction that the subject should try to make as novel a picture as possible, such that no one else will be able to produce. Elaboration is emphasized by the instruction that the subject may add as many details as he thinks necessary in order to make the picture tell as complete and as interesting a story as possible.

2. Incomplete Figures

It consists of 10 line drawings which will be made into meaningful pictures of different objects. The subject is asked to make a picture which no one else in the group will be able to think of.

3. Triangles and Ellipses

In this activity the subject is provided with 7 triangles and 7 ellipses and he is required to construct different meaningful pictures based on the two given stimuli.

The three activities taken together provide ample opportunity to the subject to use his imagination with different types of figural tasks and come out with some novel ideas.

It each activity, the picture are scored for elaboration and originality. The subject is also asked to give an interesting and suitable title to each picture. The titles may also be scored for verbal elaboration and originality and the scores added to the verbal creativity score obtained on the verbal creativity test. The scoring of the titles however is optional. Clear instructions and the time allowed for each activity are given in the test booklet itself.

Reported Psychometric Properties

Reliability

The test-retest reliabilities of the factor scores and also the total score were obtained on a rural and urban sample children (n=50). the reliabilities of factor scores and also the total creativity score were considerably high, ranging from 0.932 to 0.947. The inter-score reliabilities using 34 test scripts were found to be 0.981, 0.980 and 0.917 for elaboration, originality and total creativity scores respectively.

Validity

The validity coefficients for factor scores and total creativity score are high enough (significant at 0.01 level) to place confidence in the use of the test.

Adaptation of the Mehdi's (1973) Test of Verbal and Non-verbal Creative Thinking

The original from (English version) of Mehdi's Test of Verbal and non-verbal Creative Thinking was translated into Telugu language. The copies of both English and Telugu version were given to language experts for their comments on the translation. Their suggestions were carried out.

In the verbal test, the example of new relationship activity was modified to give more clarity. Originally man and animal were given but the investigator specified the name of the animal like cow.

Embedded Figures Test (EFT)

Due to simplicity of the material and ease of administration, the Embedded Figures Test has become the principal procedure for assessing the field dependence/ independence cognitive style.

Development of EFT

The EFT was developed by Witkin, et al (1954). The simple and complex figures which make up the EFT are modifications of figures selected from those used by Gottschaldt (1926) in his classical studies of the relative roles of contextual (field) factors and past experience in perception. In Gottschaldt's work, the sought-after simple figure was incorporated into the complex one but obscured perceptually by means of line patterns.

Preliminary experiments demonstrated that it was not possible to obtain a sufficient number of difficult figures from Gottschaldt's material, not was it possible to make up enough such figures by the use of line patterns as a means of embedding the simple figure. It therefore, became necessary to develop an additional method of obscuring the simple figures. Experimentation showed that colouring parts of the complex figures, so as to reinforce given sub-wholes, was a very effective way of making disembedding more difficult.

After extensive studies with a large series of figures and a variety of different colour arrangement 24 complex figures and 8 simple figures were selected. Each of the simple figures was embedded several different complex figures. Two main criteria were followed in selecting the complex figures. First, it was necessary to produce a series of figure graded in difficult of disembedding. Depending on the structure of the complex figure, the detection of the simple figure may be easy of difficult. Second, it was desirable to have a variety of simple figures so that no one of them would be encountered a great number of times. This was intended to reduce the role of practice.

As noted, 24 pairs of simple and complex figures were originality selected to compose the standard test. Odd-even and test-retest reliability were provided to be very satisfactory with this initial selection.

Through extensive use of the test, it was found that adequate reliability and validity could be maintained with a 12 figure test. Another way found to shorten administration time of the test, again without affecting reliability and validity, was to reduce the search time allowed per trial from 5-minutes to 3-minutes.

The test now has a 12-trial, 3-minute time limit format. The 12 figures are the first 12 of the original 24. This is Form A of the EFT. The second set of 12 figures (form B) may be used for retesting if desired.

Test Material

Cards

The test material consists of three sets of cards: two sets of 12 cards with complex figures, numbered consecutively in order of test presentation, and a set of 8 cards with simple forms, designated by letters A to H. The order of figures for test is shown below.

Form-A		Form-B	
Complex Figure	Simple Form	Complex figure	Simple form
1	A	13	E
2	B	14	C
3	C	15	D
4	D	16	G
5	E	17	A
6	A	18	E
7	F	19	B
8	E	20	C
9	C	21	G
10	G	22	A
11	A	23	E
12	H	24	C

Next to the number on the reverse side of each complex figure card is printed the letter identifying the simple form which is embedded in that complex figure. There is also one practice complex figure card (labelled P-x) and an accompanying card (labelled P) with the sample form.

The complex figure cards, each of which may be encased in a transparent plastic envelop to prolong it's life, may be bound together in numerical order in a small loose-leaf note book. A piece of transparent plastic may be placed over each card presented to the subject.

Stylus

To enable the subject to trace the outline of the simple form in each complex figure, a stylus was provided. If the user wishes, he may place a rubber tip on the end of the stylus, nevertheless, subjects should be instructed to hold the stylus just above the complex figure card and not to touch the card when tracing out the simple form.

Stop watch

A stop watch is needed with a second hand which can be stopped and restarted without resetting the hand at zero.

Reported Psychometric Properties

Reliability

Reliabilities for the 12-figure, 3 minute format are all based on data obtained by recomputing scores for tests given in the original full 24-figure, 5- minute form. All the reliabilities for the children and adolescents were computed by the Spearman-Brown method.

RELIABILITIES

Age Level	Sex	Number of Subjects	Reliability Coefficient
10 years	M	51	0.86
	F	52	0.81
11 years	M	21	0.84
	F	24	0.74
12 years	M	25	0.78
	F	25	0.74

In the present study also the split-half reliability coefficients for whole test was calculated for Sugali tribal and non-tribal children after final data collection.

RELIABILITIES

Age Level	*Sex*	*Number of Subjects*	*Reliability Coefficient*
10 years	**M**	**18**	**0.723**
	F	**17**	**0.545**
11 years	**M**	**15**	**0.623**
	F	**15**	**0.746**
12 years	**M**	**19**	**0.589**
	F	**16**	**0.670**
Non-tribal :			
10 years	**M**	**18**	**0.621**
	F	**17**	**0.527**
11 years	**M**	**15**	**0.670**
	F	**15**	**0.440**
12 years	**M**	**19**	**0.428**
	F	**16**	**0.527**

Note : M-indicates Male; F-indicates Female

Validity

A much larger literature, all used the individual EFT demonstrated the validity of the test.

Matching familiar Figures Test (MFFT)

Although many test procedures have been cited as adequate measures of the reflection-impulsivity dimensions, the technique most often used in research is the Matching Familiar Figures Test. It is a standard instrument devised by Kagan, el al (1964), to assess reflective-impulsive cognitive style in children. The literature indicates that the MFFT is valid in terms of range and structural clarity of information provided. Currently the primary deficients are a lack of norms (Thomas, Keren and George, 1981). Moreover this test may not be suitable to the Indian conditions, so the Investigator developed a MFFT depending upon the typical sample item from Kagan' test given in the book Cognitive Styles (1976).

Development of MFFT

Selection of Items

Items selected for this test were very familiar to the Sugali tribal and non-tribal children and also suitable to the local conditions. Altogether 20 items were selected. They were Flower, Brinjal, Pot, Dog, Clock, Tree, Cow, Bow and Arrow, Crow, Woman, Hut, Goat, Bicycle, School, Shop, Bore well, Boy, Hills, Bus and Sugali Woman.

Preparation of the Preliminary Test Booklet

The selected items were drawn roughly along worth five alternatives for each item. These items were given to an artist to drawn the pictures neatly and clearly. After these items were drawn they were checked thoroughly for clarity of the picture and to avoid mistakes in the pictures. All these 20 pictures were put in an order an made it as a booklet. Instructions for administration were also given in the booklet itself. Answer Sheet was also prepared.

Adapted Version of Children's Personality Questionnaire (CPQ)

The personality characteristics of creative children have been studied by a variety of techniques including (a) observational methods that utilize behaviour sampling, interviews and rating scales, (b) personality inventories such as MMPI, and (c) projective techniques, such as the Rorschach and Thematic Apperception Tests. For younger children the Early School Personality Questionnaire (6-8 years) and Children's Personality Questionnaire (8-12 years) are commonly used to asses their personality characteristics.

Description of Original Form of CPQ

The CPQ yields a general assessment of personality development by measuring fourteen distinct dimensions or traits of personality which have been found by psychologists to approach the total personality. The original form of CPQ (English version) was developed by Porter and Cattell (1972) and was first published by the Institute for Personality and Ability Testing in 1959. The test is designed to give maximum information in the shortest time about the greatest number of dimensions of personality; that are of potential importance in clinical, educational and counselling practice. The test results will help in precise and quantitative evaluation of a child's personality contributing to it's performance in schools, it's social adjustment inside and outside the classroom. The CPQ is also designed to measure both primary and second order factors according to the needs of the investigators.

The test has two published forms, form A and form B. There are 140 items in each form. Each form is further made available in two parts namely A_1; A_2 and B_1; B_2. Each part has seventy items. Each of the fourteen dimensions of personality is measured by the CPQ which has a technical name and an alphabetical symbol for convenience of reference, e.g. A, B, C, D and so forth. Each item (except the factor B-intelligence item) has a forced choice, "Yes" or "No" answer. The test is suitable for children between 8 and 12 years. Each dimension of personality is described by two extremes, low and high. The authors have recommended conversion of raw scores into standard ten scores called Stems. These score has a ten point range with a mean of 5.5 stems, of 5 and 6 represent the average or middle range. Generally, the interpretation of the test is made by drawing up a profile. Norms are provided for boys and girls separately.

Adapted Version of CPQ

The Original form of CPQ English version was adapted to Telugu language by Siddamma (1979) for research purpose. Some of the items in the original CPQ have been reworded for clarity and edited to suit the Indian way of life. The test material consists of (1) a test booklet (A_1 and A_2 forms), (2) a separate Answer Sheet, and (3) Scoring Key. The instructions, procedure for administering the test, scoring and construction of profiles etc. have not been changed in the adapted version of CPQ.

Reported Psychometric Properties

Reliability

The adapted version of the CPQ was administrated to 9^+ to 11^+ age groups (n=209) children drawn from three schools in Tirupati, Chittoor district, A.P. The Split-half reliability coefficients (corrected by Spearman-Brown formula) for form A_1 and form A_2 were 0.52 and 0.51 respectively. Therefore, it has reasonably good reliability. The stability of the test corresponds to long term test-retest correlations. The interval used here was 4 weeks. Out of the fourteen factors, eight factors namely A, C, G, H, I, J, N and O have obtained dependability coefficient of 0.7 and above. It may, therefore, be interpreted that the test has the necessary reliability and can be used in the measurement of personality characteristics of Indian children.

Rotter's (1966) Internal-External Control Scale

To asses locus of control orientation among children, a number of Internal-External-Scales have been developed in the Western countries for subjects of different ages. They are Bialer (1961) Locus of Control Scale; Crandall, at al (1965) Intellectual Achievement Responsibility Scale; Nowicki and Strickland (1973) Internal-External Control Scale and Nowicki and Duke (1974) Internal-External Control Scale. Not many serious attempts have been done by researchers to measures Internal-External Control orientation among school children in Indian set-up (Lefcourt, 1983). In the present enquiry, locus of control was measured by the Internal-External Control Scale, a 29 item test which is a revision by Liverant, Rotter and Crowne (Rotter, 1966) of an earlier 60 item instrument.

Description

Rotter's (1966) internal-External Control Scale Consists of 29 items including six filler items. These filler items are intended to make somewhat more ambiguous of the real purpose of the test. Every item is of forced-choice type. There are two sets of statements lettered a and b One of them is always worded in the external direction and is underlined. The items are so composed that they deal exclusively with subject's belief about the nature of the world, that means they are concerned with the expectations about how reinforcement is controlled. Therefore, the test is considered to be a measure of generalized expectancy. The filler items are ignored while scoring.

Reported Psychometric Properties

Reliability

Rotter (1972) reported that test data on this Internal-External Control Scale were obtained on several samples. The Internal Consistency Estimates were found reasonably high ranging from 0.65 to 0.76. Test-retest reliability for one month period also seems to be highly consistent (coefficients range from 0.49 to 0.83). Achamamba(1978) has provided information regarding the reliability of the scale for Indian sample. She has reported reliability coefficient of 0.69.

Validity

The factor analysis of this scale has been attempted. Much of the variance was found included in a general factor accounting for nearly 53 per cent of the total variance scale. Large number of studies testing the predictions in widely varying situations have indicated good discriminant validity.

Adaptation and Modification of the Items

In the present investigation, Rotter's (1966) Internal-External Control Scale was translated into Telugu, the regional language spoken by the subjects. Then it was given to a language expert with a request to examine vocabulary level, syntax and meaning. Then it was presented to five experts, each one from the fields of Education, Child Development, Anthropology and teachers of Tribal and Municipal Elementary Schools. They judged the items and ranked, 8th, 16th, 17th and 25th items, as very difficult to the sample to their level of understanding. They also suggested necessary modifications with regard to language of the items.

Adapted Version of Home Environment Inventory (HEI)

Home itself is a complex unit. The assessment of it's psychological environments is not an easy matter. Previously observation and recording of behaviours in naturally occurring environments was emphasized (Yarrow and Goodwin, 1965 and Wright, 1967). Then many significant tools like Interview Schedules were constructed for measuring parental attitudes toward child rearing (Kawash, 1968; Gibson, 1968; Sidama and Sinha 1973; Melrese, 1974; Husaini, 1975; and Kilman, 1975). Hawkes (1963) suggested that the crux of parent-child relations as far as the child in the family was concerned appeared to be in the area of children's perception of what the parents, are rather than in very children's perception of what the parents are, rather than in very definite and specific characteristics of home life; In Western countries Bronfenbrenner (1961), Mitchell (1963), Grebow (1973), Armentrout (1975), Angenent (1976), Scheck and Emerick (1976) and in India, Misra (1986) designed some of the important tools to measure children's perception of their home environment.

Description

Manjuvani and Kalyani (1987) adapted and cross validated the Misra's (1986) Home Environment Inventory for their research purpose. Hence, it was standardized on a sample of Chittoor district, A.P., the Investigator was interested to administer it in the present study with little modifications in the items.

HEI consists of one test booklet and a Response Sheet. The test booklet has two parts A and B. In the part A the items related to perceived psycho-social environment are used to give a total picture of home environment. Part B deals with physical aspects of home environment. Both part A and B together give a comprehensive behavioural, structural and experiential components of home environment.

Part A of the HEI : There are 66 items representing the 10 factors namely 1. Permissiveness, 2. Control, 3. Conformity, 4. Rejection, 5. Reward, 6. Punishment, 7. Protectiveness, 8. Nurturance, 9. Deprivation of privileges, 10. Cognitive stimulation. The operational definitions of these factors are given below:

1. **Permissiveness:** It includes provision of opportunities to child to express his views freely and act according to his desire with no interference from parents.
2. **Control:** It indicates autocratic atmosphere in which many restrictions are imposed on children by the parents in order to discipline them.
3. **Conformity:** It indicates parent's directions, commands, or orders with which child is expected to comply by action. It refers to demands to work according to parent's desires and expectations.
4. **Rejection:** It indicates hostile atmosphere which includes excessive criticism, individuals comparisons, refusal to pay attention, unconcern for the child' welfare and no right to express feelings.
5. **Reward:** It includes symbolic rewards to strengthen or increase the probability of desired behaviour.
6. **Punishment:** It implies the infliction of pain or discomfort, denial or removal of satisfaction, to eliminate the occurrence of undesirable behaviour.
7. **Protectiveness:** It implies prevention of independent behaviour and prolongation of infantile care.
8. **Nurturance:** It includes the tendency of the parents to take care of the child's physical, psychological and social re-

quirements so that the child grows happily. It involves all caring and supporting functions of the parents in a family.

9. **Deprivation of Privileges:** It implies controlling children's behaviour by taking away their rights to seek love, respect and other thing which satisfy their needs.

10. **Cognitive Stimulation:** This refers to such parental behaviour which promotes the child's awareness of its surroundings, understanding things and situations, to think and reason clearly and an overall efficiency in intelligent behaviour.

Part B of the HEI : There are 36 questions, 12 each in three categories; Availability, Opportunity and Utilization. Physical environment is evaluated taking into consideration the material facilities available, opportunity to explore them and how well they are actually utilized by the child.

Response Sheet: The subject has to write his/her background information about age, sex, number of children in the family, birth other position and standard on the Response Sheet.

In the Response Sheet, three categories of responses namely "many times" and "rarely" for Part A items and two categories of responses namely "Yes " and "No" for part B items are given. The subjects are required to mark on the Response Sheet one of the three categories for Part A (many times, some times and rarely and two categories for part B (Yes and No).

Reported Psychometric Properties

A pre-test was carried out on a sample of 120 students of 8th, 9th, and 10th standards drawn from three schools situated in Tirupati, Chittoor district, to establish basic psychometric properties of the tool. Item analysis including factor analysis was carried out. Item having poor reliability and validity were eliminated.

Reliability

The split-half (odd and even) reliability of the inventory was computed using Product Moment Coefficient of Correlation. The reliability of the half-test thus found was 0.61 When reliability of the half test boosted up using Spearman-Brown Prophecy formula, the reliability of whole test found to be 0.76. This value was considered reasonably high and therefore, was accepted.

Validity

The validity of any measuring instrument depends upon the accuracy with which it measures what it intends to measure.

Content Validity

In the construction of HEI items were selected based on careful analysis of experts. The preliminary form along with operational definitions were given to experts. They were asked to judge which dimension each item measures. An item was included under a dimension only when four or more experts included it under that dimension.

Intrinsic Validity

There is a close relationship between validity and reliability. This validity is given by the square root of the proportion of true variance. i.e., square root of it's reliability. The intrinsic validity of HEI is $\sqrt{0.76} = 0.87$.

Item Validity

The discriminative value of each statement was established by t-test and bi-serial correlation before including them in the final form.

Factor Validity

All the items included in the final form of the HEI have factor loadings of 0.03 or more. Each of the 10 factor consists of 3 or more items. Overall and Klett (1972) stated that 50 per cent to 70 per cent of the total variance was enough to consider for prediction of any psychological and psychometric domain. All the 10 factors in the present HEI put together explain 88 percent of the total variance generated by the test. Therefore, it may be regarded that the test satisfies the validity requirements. According to the instructions in test booklets and manuals all the preliminary test forms were administrated in pre-try-out and pilot study.

Pre-Try-Out

Guliford (1954) points out that a pre-try-out is the preliminary administration of the tentative try-out units to a small sample for the purpose of discovering gross deficiencies but with no intention of analyzing pre-try-out data for individual item.

Pre-try-out was carried out on 10 students of 10,11 and 12 years and (5th, 6th and 7th standards) from Tirupati, Chittoor district, A.P. to check their applicability. Students were encouraged to express their doubts freely. This enabled to locate vague items which were ambiguous or difficult to understand. Necessary further modifications were made in the light of experience gained through this pre-try-out.

Pilot Study

After exploratory study, pilot study was conducted on a sample of 30 subjects (15 Sugali tribal and 15 non-tribal) of 10,11 and 12 years (5th, 6th and 7th standards). They were drawn from Punganur Mandal of Chittoor district. Details are given in Table 3.1.

Table 3.1 : Age/Sex Distribution of Subjects Selected for Pilot-Study

Group	*Sex*	*Age*			*Total*
		10 years	*11 years*	*12 years*	(30)
Tribal	Boys	3	2	3	8
	Girls	2	3	2	7
Non-Tribal	Boys	3	2	3	8
	Girls	2	3	2	7

After administration of all the preliminary tests in pre-try-out and pilot study, the outcomes for test are as follows:

Mehdi's (1973) Test of Verbal and Non-verbal Creative Thinking

In pre-try-out and pilot study, activities in verbal and non-verbal tests of creativity were able to perform well except product improvement tasks in the Verbal Creativity Test. For that, the Investigator adapted the model of a toy, "horse" into "cat" which is more familiar one.

Embedded Figures Test

The Embedded Figures Test Form A was administered individually in pre-try-out and pilot study. The Investigator gave instructions in Telugu language for easy understanding. The subjects performed well with good understanding of instructions. So, the test is suitable to administer as it without any changes.

Matching Familiar Figures Test

The preliminary MFFT booklet was administered in pre-try-out and pilot study. According to the instructions given in the test booklet, it was given to each child individually in Telugu regional language. After completion of the pilot study, 30 Answer Sheets were scored by giving 1 mark for each correct response.

Item Analysis

Item analysis provides some safeguards against inclusion of irrelevant items. Guliford (1954) and Garrett (1981) have favoured employing item analysis for improving the reliability and validity of a test. Item analysis is essential to know that percentage of the group is able to answer the item and how difficult the items is whether the item is able to discriminate the high scoring individual from the low scoring individual and whether the distractors are effectively functioning.

The Answer Sheets from the pilot study were arranged in an ascending order of sores with lowest score at the bottom and highest score at the top. Fro this, top 27 per cent and bottom 27 per cent of the Answer Sheets were selected and formed the upper criterion group (UCG) and lower criterion group (LCG). Number and percentage of right responses in the top 27 per cent (UCG) and number and percentage of right responses in the bottom 27 per cent (LCG) were calculated. Then facility Value of item which is statistical measure of item difficulty was calculated by the formula which as follows:

$$\text{Facility Value of Item} = \frac{\text{Number of individuals answering the item correctly}}{\text{Total number of individuals}}$$

An item which had Facility Value of 0.35 to 0.85 was retained and less than 0.35 (low score) was deleted because those items were difficult items. The Difficulty Index of each item was also found by averaging the percents correct in the UCG and LCG. Validity or Discrimination Index of each item was found by using Flanagan's table of normalized bi-serial coefficients. According to Garrett (1981) items with validity indices of 0.20 or more regarded as satisfactory and the items are good enough to differentiate the high from the low scores on a test.

Totally two items (15th and 19th) were deleted which were very difficult and had no validity. They were shop and bus. Finally 18 items were retained in the final booklet. To see whether the distractions were effectively functioning, the Distractor Analysis was done and it was satisfactory.

Preparation of the Final Test Booklet

All these 18 items were arranged in an order to difficulty and they were made into a booklet form. Once again the Answer Sheet was prepared.

Adapted Version of Children's Personality Questionnaire

The adapted version of CPQ was administered in pre-try-out and pilot study sample following the standard procedure and instructions given in test booklet and manual. Due to unfamiliarity of language to the sample, some of the items (26th and 49th in form A_1 and 30th, 49th and 61st in form A_2) were not answered by the subjects. That is why the Investigator modified the Telugu language of these items without any change in the meaning.

Rotter's (1966) Internal-External Control Scale

When Rotter's (1961) Internal-External Control Scale was administered in the pre-try-out and pilot study, the same items which were ranked by experts as very difficult were not responded by the subjects. Garrett and Woodworth (1965) stated that the difficulty of an item might be determined in several ways: (1) by the judgement of competent people who rank the items in order of difficulty, (2) by how quickly the item can be solved, and (3) by the number examinees in the group who get the item right. The Investigator deleted those items which were very difficult from the Rotter's Internal-External Control Scale. Finally the Rotter's Internal-External Control Scale contained 25 items including five filler items. There was no change with regard to instructions for administration.

Adapted Version of Home Environment Inventory

The preliminary form of adapted version of HEI was administered in pre-try-out and pilot study in order to get feedback regarding understandability of instructions and the items by the students. This experience was helpful in effecting necessary modifications to the language of the statements. The modification and improvements were carried out wherever necessary, in order to ensure the clarity.

SAMPLE FOR FINAL STUDY

The location of the study area is the Chittoor district. This district comes under Rayalaseema region of Andhra Pradesh and it is agriculturally, economically and socially backward. The Chittoor district is comprised of 66 newly constituted Mandals.

For the purpose of the study, at the first stage the Investigator purposively selected three Mandals from Chittoor namely Phunganur, Madanapalli and Piler. The different criteria governing the selection of these Mandals are as follows:

1. The Sugali tribals residing in these Mandals are a representative sample of the group in Chittoor district.
2. It's closeness to Tirupati from where the investigator had to carry out the research.
3. Convenience in reaching.

In the second stage, the Investigator conducted exploratory study to know more details about the sample. In the exploratory study it was observed the Sugalis mostly residing in the certain villages of each Mandal have separate tribal schools. Based on those findings, the Investigator selected two villages-one for Sugali tribal and an other for non-tribal sample children from each Mandal. Non-tribal villages means surrounding villages of Sugalis where only non-Sugali tribal population was studied. The total population and scheduled tribe population in each Mandal and the selected villages in each Mandal are given in Table 3.2

After collecting the total population of Sugali tribal children and non-tribal children in the selected villages, the Investigator chose a comparable group of 100 Sugali tribal and 199 non-tribal sample children of both sexes representing 10,11 and 12 years age group. Based on age and sex, the sample was selected by using the Stratified Random Sampling Method. Moreover, these age group children (10,11 and 12 years) were found studying 5th, 6th and 7th standards respectively in Tribal and Municipal Elementary Schools. Table 3.3 shows the age/sex distribution of the sample of the final study.

Details about Population and Selected Villages in the Mandals

(According to 1981 Census)

Name of the Mandal	*Total Population*	*Scheduled Tribe Population*	*Selected Villages*	
			Sugali-tribal	Non-tribal
Punganur	63,337	2,239	Sugali-mitta	Ragani-palli
Madanappali	1,00,614	3,171	Ankki-setti Palli	Pappi Reddy Gari Palli
Piler	39,749	1,648	Jandla	Mudupula Vemula

Table 3.3 : Age/Sex Distribution of the Sample Children for Final Study

Age Groups	*Sugali tribal children*		*Non-tribal children*	
	Boys	*Girls*	*Boys*	*Girls*
10 years	18	17	18	17
11 years	15	15	15	15
12 years	19	16	19	16
Total	**52**	**48**	**52**	**48**

DATA COLLECTION

After securing permission from the Head-master/Head-mistress in each of the selected schools, necessary arrangements were made in the schools for the selection of samples and administration of the tests. Before administering the tests to the respondents, an effort were made to establish rapport with them. The purpose of the administration of the tests was explained to each subject well in advance. The required data were collected by the investigator from the subjects directly through the administration of different tests prepared for the purpose. Care was taken to make the subject respond all the items in the tests without hesitation.

Administration

The tests viz,. Mehdi's (1973) Test of Verbal and Non-verbal

Creative Thinking, (adapted by the Investigator), EFT, MFFT (developed by the Investigator), adapted version of CPQ (modified by the Investigator, Rotter's (1966) Internal-External Control Scale (adapted and modified by the Investigator), adapted version of HEI (Modified by the Investigator) were administered according to the procedure and instructions given in test booklets and manuals.

The total time taken for data collection was four months (including exploratory and pilot study).

SCORING OF THE INSTRUMENTS

Mehdi's (1973) Test of Verbal and Non-Verbal Creative Thinking

Based on the procedure given in manuals for scoring in verbal tests of creativity, the new scores for each activity and total for fluency, flexibility and originality components were obtained. Based on the procedure for scoring in non-verbal tests of creativity, the raw scores for each activity and total for elaboration and originality components were obtained. The scores for titles were also analyzed as explained in the manual.

The total raw scores for fluency, flexibility, originality of verbal creativity and elaboration and originality of non-verbal creativity was converted into "T" scores.

After converting the standard "T" scores in the absence of norms for tribals and non-tribals sample of particular age groups, the interpretation had to be based on high and low scores in the tests. The scores which were 1 SD above the mean were used to mark out the 'high creative' group, and those which were 1 SD below the mean were used to designate the 'low creative' group. Middle, ones were 'average creative' group.

Embedded Figure Test

The time of solution for each item was converted into seconds and recorded in the last column on the Data Sheet. Failed items were entered as 180 seconds. The solution times for the 12 items were summed and divided by 12. The resulting value, which was the mean solution time per item, was the subject's score for the test. Mean ±1 SD were used as criteria to mark the field dependents and field independents. Mean ±1 SD above scores (54.62) were considered as field dependents and below scores (52.62) as field independents.

Middle ones were unclassified.

Matching Familiar Figures Test

Most of the investigators used latency and error scores for identifying reflectives and impulsives using a traditional cut off point in the distribution of scores. The existing methodology to assess reflection/impulsivity dimension has been criticized on many grounds (Block, Block and Harrington, 1974). In order to check whether an alternative possibility which would yield a better measure as index making use of right and wrong responses along with the median split of latency was strived on the data. The results of this attempt have revealed a consistent pattern of the distribution of the subjects.

In the Answer Sheet the right and wrong responses were recorded for each subject. The time taken to give the first response (latency) was also recorded for each item. For each subject therefore, there will be number of right and wrong responses and latency score (total time in seconds over the items).

The following Reflection/Impulsivity (R-I) index was used to find out the score of each individual

$$R-I=\frac{\text{Right responses}-\text{Wrong responses}}{\text{Right responses}+\text{Wrong responses}}$$

The latency median value was 189.5 seconds.

The subjects who obtained R–I index scores 0 to 1.0 and fall above the latency median value were classified as reflectives. The subjects who obtained R–I index scores –0.1 to–1.0 and fall below the latency median value were classified as impulsives.

The subjects who got R-I index scores 0.89 and above up to 1.0 were classified as fast and accurates. The subjects who obtained R-I index scores —0.89 and above up —1.0 were classified as slow and inaccurates. For the latency the double median split procedure was used.

The correlation coefficient between R-I index scores and latency was calculated i.e., 0.64 which indicates positive correlation.

In the present study only three groups, reflectives, impulsives and slow and inaccurates were identified.

Adapted Version of CPQ

As per the manual and scoring key, the responses to the questionnaire were scored. Raw scores were found for each factor separately. The stem equivalents are to be read off from a table giving the raw scores and corresponding stem scores.

The two extremes of the factor low and high indicate the personality of the individual separately.

Rotter's (1966) Internal-External Control Scale

The test was scored by counting the number of statements out of 20 selected by an individual which was underlined. Thus, the maximum possible score was 20. The higher the score of an individual the greater is his/her externality in the control of reinforcement.

The median value was calculated for the obtained scores. The median value was 9.273. Scores below the median value were considered internal. Rotter (1966) also reported that internals were defined as subjects obtaining a score of 9 or below on Rotter's Scale.

Adapted Version of HEI

Part A: The numerical values of 3, 2 and 1 were assigned corresponding to the many times, sometimes and rarely categories and this order of weightage reversed in case of negative items. After entering the scores of all items on Response Sheets, scores of various items belonging to a specific factor were added up. thus, ten composite scores corresponding to the ten factors were available for each subject.

Part B: One mark assigned to "Yes" responses and zero to "No" responses. After having scored all the questions, scores obtained by each subjected on availability, opportunity and utilization were added separately.

The total home environment score for each subject could be obtained by summing the scores of ten part A factors. The higher the score, the better the home environment is. In part B, three scores, one on each availability, opportunity and utilization could be obtained. The higher the scores, the higher is the availability, opportunity and utilization. To make best use of the available data it was decided to interpret basic on magnitude of some key items.

STATISTICAL TECHNIQUES USED IN THE STUDY

— Number of children showing different levels of creativity and different cognitive styles in tribal and non-tribal group were given through percentages. Chi-square analysis was also carried out in necessary aspects.

— The difference between tribal and non-tribal children on dependent and independent variables was studies through t-test and f-test.

— The relationship between the two dependent variables (creativity and cognitive styles) was also found by Correlation Coefficients.

— Two series of Multiple, Regression Analysis were done, one regression upon creativity, the other on cognitive style as dependent variables. The age, sex, locus of control, total home environment were independent variables. The inter-correlation with dependent variable in tribal and non-tribal group were also calculated.

— Personality profiles were also drawn to see the personality characteristics of individuals, fitting into different levels of creativity and cognitive styles. The Profile Similarity Coefficient (r_p) value was also calculated.

— The Discriminant Function analysis was use to see whether tribal and non-tribal children fall correctly in their categories based on the variables' scores.

— In the next chapter the results of the analysis are presented systematically together with relevant interpretations within the scope of the main objectives of the study.

4

RESULTS AND DISCUSSION

In this chapter the results are presented and discussed systematically in six sections as noted below:

1. The first section deals with the number of Children showing different levels of creativity and different cognitive styles in tribal and non-tribal group through Percentages. In this, the degree of association between high, average and low creatives and components of creativity in tribal and non-tribal group, the association between cognitive styles and tribal and non-tribal community are also through chi-square analysis.
2. In the second section, the difference between tribal and non-tribal children on the scores of dependent and indepen-.ent variables were presented through t-test and F-test.
3. The third section deals with the relationship between creativity and cognitive styles in tribal and non-tribal children through correlation coefficients.
4. The results of the Multiple (step-wise) Regression Analysis, along with inter-correlations among independent variables and their correlation with dependent variable in tribal and non-tribal group are reported in the fourth section.
5. In the fifth section, Personality Profiles are drawn according to different levels of creativity and different cognitive styles. The Profile Similarity Coefficient (rp) value was

also calculated to see the similarity/dissimilarity of the personality of tribal and non-tribal children.

6. The results of the Discriminant function Analysis to establish the contributions of the variables to classify the tribal and non-tribal children are presented in the sixth section.

1. NUMBER OF CHILDREN SHOWING DIFFERENT LEVELS OF CREATIVITY AND DIFFERENT COGNITIVE STYLES IN TRIBAL AND NON-TRIBAL GROUPS

Number of Children Showing Different Levels of Creativity

In the present study verbal and non-verbal creativity in Sugali tribal and non-tribal children was measured. The raw creativity scores were converted into standard scores and criterion groups, high, average and low creative children were identified on the basis of ±1 SD from the mean.

The percentage of high, average and low creative on verbal and non-verbal components of creativity in tribal and non-tribal groups are shown in Table 4.1.

Table 4.1 : Percentage Incidence of Creative Children in Tribal and Non-tribal Groups

Group	*Components of Creativity*	*High Creatives*	*Average Creatives*	*Low Creatives*	*X^2 Values*
Tribal (n=100)	Verbal	42	10	48	0.22 NS
	Non-Verbal	43	10	47	
Non-tribal (n=100)	Verbal	49	9	42	1.862 NS
	Non-Verbal	43	6	51	

NS = Not Significant

The total sample consists of 100 Sugali and 100 non-tribal children. Among them 42 per cent and 49 per cent are high creatives in verbal components of creativity respectively. The equal number (43 per cent) of children in tribal and non-tribal group are high creatives in non-verbal components of creativity.

With regard to average creative in verbal creativity. 10 per cent of tribal and 9 per cent of non-tribal children are identified. Ten percent of tribal and 6 per cent of non-tribal children are considered average creatives in non-verbal creativity.

Whereas low creatives are considered, 48 per cent of tribal and 42 per cent of non-tribal children in verbal creativity and 47 per cent of tribal and 51 per cent of non-tribal children in non-verbal creativity are classified as low creatives.

From the above findings it is clear that a relatively high percentage of non-tribal children are identified as high creatives in verbal creativity when compared to tribal children. In other words the tribal children are deficient in regard to the level of verbal creative thinking. The reason being the disadvantages from an early age. In deprived homes, working class parents depend heavily on "restricted code" through which thoughts are communicated in a limited, condensed way lacking precise conceptualization and differentiation. With the result that the interacting of social interaction on the basis of restricted languages helps vigorously in retarding child's speech and thought processes.

Koske (1977) reported that parents of tribal children talk very little with their children. They talk in their dialect which has a small vocabulary not exceeding 300 words. So the disadvantaged child's cognitive abilities are not fully developed and he is usually unable to meet the challenge of school and take full advantage of the educational facilities offered at a latter stage (Narmada, 1972).

With regard to non-verbal creativity the equal number of high creativity are identified in tribal and non-tribal children. That means tribal children's performance in non-verbal creative measures is similar to the non-tribal children's performance. Non-verbal creative tests, being tests of finger manipulation, probably appealed to tribal children also. Some creative children have difficulty in expressing their ideas in writing. They are in a better position to express their ideas in the form of figures.

In order to explore the strength of association between high, average and low creative and verbal and non-verbal components of creativity in tribal and non-tribal children, chi-square (X^2) analysis was carried out. The analysis reveals that there is no significant association between high, average and low creatives and verbal and non-verbal creativity in tribal ($X^2 = 0.22$, df = 2) and non-tribal ($X^2 = 1.862$, df = 2) children.

According to age and sex, the percentage incidence of creatives in tribal and non-tribal children in given in Table 4.2 and 4.3 respectively.

Table 4.2 shows that 50 per cent of tribal boys in the 10 years age group are high creatives in verbal creativity. Whereas the other 50 per cent of them are low creatives. On the other hand, in non-verbal components of creativity, 61.11 per cent of boys in this age groups are considered to be low creatives. When girls are taken into account more percentage of tribal girls (41.18 per cent) fall under average creatives in verbal creativity. Whereas in non-verbal creativity, their percentage (47.06 per cent) is more in low creatives category.

In 11 years age group, more than half of the tribal boys are high creatives in verbal (53.33 per cent) as well as non-verbal (53.33 per cent) components of creativity. On the other hand, 53.3 per cent and 46.67 percent of girls fall under low creatives in verbal and non-verbal creativity respectively.

Higher percentage of the tribals boys (57.89 per cent) in 12 years age groups are classified as low creatives in verbal creativity. Whereas similar number of boys (47.37 per cent) have demonstrated to be high as well as low creatives in non-verbal creativity. When girls are taken into consideration, equal number of them fall under high and low creatives in verbal creativity. In non-verbal creativity 50 per cent of the girls shows high creativity whereas 43.75 per cent low creatives.

From this analysis it is clear that many of the tribal boys with 11 years age are classified as high creatives in verbal and non-verbal components of creativity. Whereas many of the tribal girls in the same age group have exhibited low creatives in verbal and non-verbal creativity.

Table 4.3 indicates that more than half of the non-tribal boys (55.55 per cent) in 10 years age groups are categories as high creatives in verbal components of creativity. Further, it also reveals that 61.11 per cent of boys shows low creatives in non-verbal creativity. On the other hand, 47.06 per cent of the non-tribal girls in this age groups are considered high creatives in verbal components of creativity. Whereas equal number of them fall under high (47/06 per cent) and low (47.06

Table 4.2 : Percentage Incidence of Creative Children in Tribal Group by Age and Sex

Age Level	*Components of Creativity*	*High Creatives*		*Average Creatives*		*Low Creatives*	
		Boys	*Girls*	*Boys*	*Girls*	*Boys*	*Girls*
10 Years (n=35) (B=18+G=17)	Verbal	9 (50.00)	4 (23.53)	--	7 (41.18)	9 (50.00)	6 (35.29)
	Non-verbal	6 (33.33)	7 (41.18)	1 (5.55)	2 (11.76)	11 (61.11)	8 (47.06)
11 Years (n=30) (B=15+G=15)	Verbal	8 (53.33)	6 (40.00)	--	1 (6.67)	7 (46.67)	8 (53.33)
	Non-verbal	8 (53.33)	5 (33.33)	2 (13.33)	3 (20.00)	5 (33.33)	7 (46.67)
12 Years (n=35) (B=19+G=16)	Verbal	8 (42.11)	7 (43.75)	--	2 (12.50)	11 (57.89)	7 (43.75)
	Non-verbal	9 (47.37)	8 (50.00)	1 (5.26)	1 (6.25)	9 (47.37)	7 (43.75)

Note : Percentages are indicated in parantheses. B=Boys G=Girls.

Table 4.3 : Percentage Incidence of Creative Children in Non-Tribal Group by Age and Sex

Age Level	*Components of Creativity*	*High Creatives*		*Average Creatives*		*Low Creatives*	
		Boys	*Girls*	*Boys*	*Girls*	*Boys*	*Girls*
10 Years (n=35)	Verbal	10 (55.55)	8 (47.06)	--	2 (11.76)	8 (44.44)	7 (41.18)
(B=18+G=17)	Non-verbal	7 (38.88)	8 (47.06)	--	1 (5.88)	11 (61.11)	8 (47.06)
11 Years (n=30)	Verbal	7 (46.67)	5 (33.33)	--	2 (13.33)	8 (53.33)	8 (53.33)
(B=15+G=15)	Non-verbal	6 (40.00)	6 (40.00)	2 (13.33)	1 (6.67)	7 (46.67)	8 (53.33)
12 Years (n=35)	Verbal	11 (57.89)	8 (50.00)	1 (5.26)	4 (25.00)	7 (36.84)	4 (25.00)
(B=19+G=16)	Non-verbal	9 (47.37)	7 (43.75)	2 (10.53)	--	8 (42.10)	9 (56.25)

Note : Percentages are indicated in parantheses. B=Boys G=Girls.

per cent) creative categories in non-verbal creativity.

In 11 years age group, many of the non-tribal boys are found to be low creatives in verbal boys are found to be low creatives in verbal (53.33 per cent) and non-verbal (46.67 per cent) components of creativity. Similarly, 53.33 per cent of the girls exhibited low creativity in verbal and non-verbal components of creativity.

Most of the non-tribal boys in 12 years age groups are found to be high creative in verbal (57.89 per cent) and non-verbal (47.37 per cent) creativity. On the other hand, 50 per cent of the girls fall under high creativity in verbal and 56.25 per cent under low creatives in non-verbal creativity.

From the above findings it is found that in the non-verbal 11 years age group, many of the boys and girls are classified as low creatives in verbal and non-verbal creativity. Many of the non-tribal boys with 12 years age are identified as high creatives in verbal and non-verbal components of creativity. Half of the girls in this age showed high creatives in verbal and more than half as low creatives in non-verbal components of creativity.

Number of Children Showing Different Cognitive Styles

The percentage of children showing field dependence/independence and reflection/impulsivity cognitive styles in tribal and non-tribal children are given in Table 4.4.

Among the total Sugali tribal sample (n = 100), 51 per cent are filed dependents, 41 per cent field independents and 8 per cent unclassified group children.

It is also observed that in total non-tribal sample (n = 100) 42 per cent are field dependents, 55 per cent field independents and 3 per cent considered unclassified group children.

With regard to reflection/ impulsivity cognitive style, 8 per cent are classified as reflectives, 91 per cent as impulsives and 1 per cent as slow and inaccurates in tribal group. In the non-tribal group, 12 per cent of them are identified as reflectives, 84 per cent as impulsives and the remaining 4 per cent as slow and inaccurates.

From the above findings, it is observed that a higher percentage of tribal children are field dependents. Dershowtiz (1971) reported that field-dependence cognitive style is functionally related to cultural

Table 4.4 : Percentage of Children Showing Cognitive Styles in Tribal and Non-tribal Group

Group	*Field Dependence/Independence Cognitive Style*			X^2 Value	*Reflection/Impulsivity Cognitive Style*			X^2 Value
	Field dependents	*Field indepen-dents*	*Unclassi-fied*		*Reflec-tives*	*Impul-sives*	*Slow and inaccu-rates*	
Tribal (n=100)	51	41	8	5.184 NS	8	91	1	2.88 NS
Non-tribal (n=100)	42	55	3		12	84	4	

patterns which emphasize the maintenance of traditional order. As most of the tribal communities come under undifferentiated traditional societies, the field dependence cognitive style is commonly seen in tribal children.

It is also noticed that relatively higher percentage of non-trial children are filed independents. Dershowitz (1971) reported that those manifesting high levels in field independence are more characteristically found in complex, modern and industrialized societies. Tharakan (1987) also reported that subjects reside in urban environments are relatively more field independents and individual's levels of independence is positively related to the levels of economic development, modernization and industrialization influences. It is examined in the present study that non-tribal children have more influence to urbanization and industrialization when compared to tribal children who are more field independents.

To know the degree of association between cognitive styles (field dependence/independence and reflection/impulsivity) and tribal and non-tribal community, X^2-analysis was employed. The analysis reveals that there is no statistically significant association between field dependents, field independents and unclassified and tribal and non-tribal groups ($X^2 = 5.184$, df = 2). Also, It is noticed that there is no significant association between reflectives, impulsives and slow and inaccurates and tribal and non-tribal groups ($X^2 = 2.88$, df = 2).

According to age and sex the percentage of children showing field dependence/independence cognitive style in tribal and non-tribal group are presented in Table 4.5 and 4.6 respectively.

Table 4.5 reveals that a higher percentage of tribal boys (83.33 per cent) girls (88.23 per cent) in 10 years age group are field dependents. Only 16.67 per cent of boys and 11.76 per cent of girls are field independents.

In 11 years age, 46.67 per cent of tribal boys are field dependents, 20 per cent field independent and 33.33 per cent unclassified group. As far as the tribal girls are concerned, it is noticed that many (80 per cent) of them are field dependents and a few (13.33 per cent) are field independents.

It is of interest to note that majority of the tribal boys (94.7 per cent) and girls (81.25 per cent) in 12 years age group are found to be

Table 4.5 : Percentage of Children Showing Field Development/ Independence Cognitive Style in Tribal Group by Age and Sex

Age Level	*Field Dependents*		*Field Independents*		*Unclassified*	
	Boys	Girls	Boys	Girls	Boys	Girls
10 years (n = 35)	15 (83.33)	15 (88.23)	3 (16.67)	2 (11.76)	--	--
11 Years (n = 30)	7 (46.67)	12 (80.00)	3 (20.00)	2 (13.33)	5 (33.33)	1 (6.67)
12 Years (n = 35)	--	2 (12.50)	18 (94.74)	13 (81.25)	1 (5.26)	1 (6.25)

Note : Percentages are indicated in parentheses.

field independents.

From the above findings, it is noticed that many of the tribal boys and girls are field dependents 10 years age. In 11 years age groups, the percentage of field dependents in boys and girls are decreased when compared to 10 years age group. Higher percentage of boys and girls are seen as filed independents in 12 years age group.

The data presented in Table 4.6 shows that in 10 years age group, a higher percentage of non-tribal boys (88.89 per cent) and girls (98.12 per cent) are found to be field dependents and the remaining as independents.

Whereas in 11 years age group, more than half of the non-tribal sample boys (66.67 per cent) and girls (53.33 per cent) are classified as field independents when compared to field dependents and unclassified group.

It is also clear that almost all the non-tribal boys (100 per cent) and girls (93.75 per cent) in 12 years age groups are field independents.

From this analysis it is found that most of the non-tribal boys and girls are field dependents in 10 years age group. More than half of the boys and girls are field-independents in 11 years age group. In the 12 years age group greater percentage is considered to be field independents.

Table 4.6 : Percentage of Children Showing Field Dependence/ Independence Cognitive Style in Non-tribal Group by Age and Sex

Age Level	*Field Dependents*		*Field Independents*		*Unclassified*	
	Boys	**Girls**	**Boys**	**Girls**	**Boys**	**Girls**
10 years (n = 35)	16 (88.89)	16 (94.12)	2 (11.11)	1 (5.88)	--	--
11 Years (n = 30)	3 (20.00)	6 (40.00)	10 (66.67)	8 (53.33)	2 (13.33)	1 (6.67)
12 Years (n = 35)	--	1 (6.25)	19 (100.00)	15 (93.75)	--	--

Note : Percentages are indicated in parentheses.

Most of the girls in 10 and 11 years age from tribal and non-tribal groups (Table 4.5 and 4.6 are found to be field dependents.) Witkin, et al (1974) demonstrated that women of any given society are more field dependent than men. Women manifest a uniformly field dependent cognitive style across sub-cultures and appear to support the contention that the universal cultural expectations and the biological role of women predisposes them to be relatively field dependent.

The similar finding is observed in tribal and non-tribal groups i.e., when age increases the percentage of children with field independence cognitive style is mostly seen. Moreover, higher percentage of boys are field independents when compared to girls. This findings is in line with Crandall and Sinkeldam (1964) and Hus and Kayson (1985) studies where the results showed that age and sex are significant that elders and boys exhibited more field independence than youngers and girls.

This finding is supported also by Miller (1953). Gump (1955) Zuckman (1957), Bieri, Bradburn and Galinsky (1958), Young (1959), and Witkin, et al (1962), reported that males are more field independent and more articulative than females. This may be due to the result of socialization process which tends to make males more field independent and females more field dependent (Witkin, et al., 1974).

According to age and sex the percentage of reflection/impulsivity cognitive style in tribal and non-tribal children are presented in Table 4.7 and 4.8 respectively.

Table 4.7 : Percentage of Children Showing Reflection/ Impulsivity Cognitive Style in Tribal Group by Age and Sex

Age Level	Reflectives		Impulsives		Slow and Inaccurates	
	Boys	Girls	Boys	Girls	Boys	Girls
10 years (n = 35)	1 (5.55)	1 (5.88)	17 (94.44)	15 (88.23)	--	1 (5.88)
11 Years (n = 30)	1 (6.67)	3 (20.00)	14 (93.33)	12 (80.00)	--	--
12 Years (n = 35)	1 (5.26)	1 (6.25)	18 (94.74)	15 (93.75)	--	--

An analysis of Table 4.7 reveals that in 10 years age group, very few of the tribal boys (5.55 per cent) and girls (5.88 per cent) are classified as reflectives. A majority of the boys (94.44 per cent) and girls (88.23 per cent) are categorised as impulsives. Only 5.88 per cent of girls are found to be slow and inaccurates.

In 11 years age tribal children group, only 6.67 per cent of boys and 20 per cent of girls are reflectives. Most of the boys (93.33 per cent) and girls (80 per cent) are found to be impulsives.

Very few tribal boys (5.26 per cent) and girls (6.25 per cent) are classified as reflectives in 12 years age level and many of the boys (94.74 per cent) and girls (93.75 per cent) are considered as impulsives.

From the above findings it is observed that irrespective of age very few tribal boys and girls are classified as reflectives. Most of the boys and girls are found to be impulsives in 10 years and 12 years age group when compared to 11 years age group.

An examination of Table 4.8 shows that none of the non-tribal boys and girls in 10 years age group are found to be respectives. A majority of boys (94.44 per cent) and girls (94.12 per cent) are considered as impulsives. Only 5.55 per cent of boys and 5.88 per cent of girls are classified as slow and inaccurates.

With reference to 11 years age non-tribal children, only 6.67 per cent of boys and 13.33 per cent of girls are reflectives. Most of the boys (80 per cent) and girls (86.67 per cent) are classified as impulsives and 13.33 per cent of boys slow anu inaccurates.

Table 4.8 : Percentage of Children Showing Reflection/Impulsivity Cognitive Style in Non-Tribal Group by Age and Sex

Age Level	*Reflectives*		*Impulsives*		*Slow and Inaccurates*	
	Boys	Girls	Boys	Girls	Boys	Girls
10 years (n = 35)	--	--	17 (94.44)	16 (94.12)	1 (5.55)	1 (5.88)
11 Years (n = 30)	1 (6.67)	2 (13.33)	12 (80.00)	13 (86.67)	3 (13.33)	--
12 Years (n = 35)	4 (21.05)	5 (31.25)	15 (78.95)	11 (68.75)	--	--

Among 12 years age non-tribal children group, 21.05 per cent of boys and 31.25 per cent of girls are identified as reflectives whereas 78.95 per cent of boys and 68.75 per cent of girls impulsives.

From the results, it is evident that in the 12 years age non-tribal group, the reflectives are found to be more in number when compared to 11 years age non-tribal groups. In other words, when age increases the presence of reflection cognitive style also increases and impulsivity cognitive style decreases. Research indicates a tendency among children to become more reflective with increase in age (Ault, 1973; Campbell and Douglas, 1972; Fancher, 1969, Kagan, 1965; Ward, 1973; and Salkind and Nelson, 1980)

2. THE DIFFERENCE BETWEEN TRIBAL AND NON-TRIBAL CHILDREN ON DEPENDENT AND INDEPENDENT VARIABLES SCORES

In this study, creativity (verbal and non-verbal) and cognitive styles (field dependence/independence and reflection/ impulsivity) are the dependent variables and the major independent variables are the personality, locus of control and home environment. Both for the scores of dependent and independent variables of tribal and non-tribal children, means, standard deviations and to or values are presented across age and sex.

It is evident from Table 4.9 that under verbal creativity, fluency, flexibility, originality and elaboration components were examined. The total score of four components was also calculated. The mean scores of fluency flexibility, originality and elaboration components

Table 4.9 : Mean, Standard Deviation (in parentheses) of Components of Verbal and Non-verbal Creativity Scores in a Sample of Children and t-Values

Components of Creativity	*Sample of Children (N=200)* Tribal (n=100)	Non-Tribal (n=100)	t	P
Verbal				
Fluency	11.440 (6.466)	14.410 (6.815)	3.161	<0.01
Flexibility	7.700 (4.850)	9.420 (5.819)	2.270	<0.05
Originality	8.520 (5.421)	11.950 (6.316)	4.121	<0.01
Elaboration	7.400 (4.295)	8.860 (3.977)	2.494	<0.05
Total Score	35.050 (18.622)	44.650 (20.325)	3.483	<0.01
Non-verbal				
Elaboration	18.540 (7.992)	18.150 (6.899)	0.369	NS
Originality	9.480 (3.647)	9.120 (2.868)	0.582	NS
Total Score	28.020 (10.467)	27.270 (8.779)	0.549	NS

of tribal children are 11.4, 7.7, 8.52 and 7.4 respectively and the mean scores of non-tribal children for the same components are 14.41, 9.42, 11.95 and 8.86 respectively. The mean scores of total components of verbal creativity in verbal and non-tribal children are 35.05 and 44.65 respectively. The value of "t" test which was used to test the difference between two group was found to be significant which shows that non-tribal children excel the tribal children in verbal components of creativity. The similar finding was observed by Krishnakumari, Lalitha and Paramaji (1986).

Under non-verbal creativity, elaboration and originality components were studied. The total score of two components was also examined. The mean scores of elaboration and originality components of tribal children are 18.54 and 9.48 and for non-tribal children 18.15 and 9.21 respectively. The mean scores of total components of non-verbal creativity in tribal and non-tribal children are 28.02 and 27.27 respectively. The "t" value indicates that there is no significant difference between tribal and non-tribal children with regard to non-verbal creativity.

It is apparent from Table 4.10 that the total components of verbal creativity mean scores for 10,11 and 12 years tribal children are 26.143, 30.4 and 47.943 respectively. On the other hand, the mean score of the total components of verbal creativity for 10,11 and 12 years in non-tribal groups are 35.457 , 33.9 and 63.057 respectively.

In tribal group, the mean score of the total components of non-verbal creativity for 10,11 and 12 years are 21,657, 27.633 and 34.714 respectively. Whereas in non-tribal group, the mean scores for the same age group are 22.571, 25.668 and 33.343 respectively.

The F-values shows that the difference in performance between the successive age groups is significant for all verbal and non-verbal components of creative measure in tribal and non-tribal children. These differences are significant at 0.01 level.

A close examination of this Table reveals several interesting points. In tribal group, when age increased the verbal and non-verbal components of creativity also increased. This finding was substantiated by Piers, et al. (1960), Raina (1970) and Venkata Rami Reddy and Saleema (1988) who studied non-tribals and revealed that creativity scores increases with the chronological age.

Whereas in non-tribal group, 11 years of age group children showed lower level of performance, than that of the 10 years age group in all verbal components of creativity except elaboration (7.60) component. In non-verbal creativity, only originality component showed lower level of performance than the 10 years age group. This result is supported by Torrance (1964) that creative abilities decline between sixth and seventh grades.

On the whole, the 12 years age group gets the highest mean values in verbal and non-verbal components of creativity in tribal and non-tribal children.

Table 4.11 reveals that the mean score of the total components of verbal creativity in tribal group is 42.0 for boys and 27.52 for girls.With regard to non-tribalchildren, the mean score of the total components of verbal creativity for boys and girls are 49.788 and 39.083 respectively.

Table 4.10 : Mean, Standard Deviation (in parentheses) of Components of Verbal and Non-verbal Creativity Scores of 10, 11 and 12 years Age Group in a Sample of Children and F-Values

	COMPONENTS OF CREATIVITY							
	Verbal					*Non-verbal*		
	Fluency	*Flexibility*	*Originality*	*Elaboration*	*Total Score*	*Elaboration*	*Originality*	*Total Score*
TRIBAL (n=100) **Age Groups**								
10 years (n = 35)	8.943 (5.241)	6.200 (3.969)	5.943 (3.780)	5.057 (3.910)	26.143 (14.309)	13.657 (7.008)	8.000 (3.281)	21.657 (9.213)
11 years (n=30)	10.800 (5.950)	7.167 (4.639)	6.433 (4.116)	6.033 (3.232)	30.400 (16.338)	19.433 (8.207)	8.200 (3.022)	27.633 (10.139)
12 years (n=35)	14.486 (6.908)	9.657 (5.280)	12.885 (5.149)	10.914 (3.081)	47.943 (17.476)	20.657 (6.058)	12.057 (3.105)	34.714 (7.649)
F	7.5151	5.094	26.593	28.086	17.870	14.454	18.125	18.459
P	<0.01	<0.01	<0.01	<0.01	<0.01	<0.01	<0.01	<0.01
NON-TRIBAL (n=100) **Age Groups**								
10 years (n=35)	12.600 (5.163)	7.200 (3.445)	9.314 (4.028)	6.343 (3.189)	34.457 (12.227)	14.429 (6.199)	8.114 (2.494)	22.571 (7.469)
11 years (n=30)	11.033 (4.414	6.800 (3.274)	8.433 (3.370)	7.600 (2.415)	33.900 (10.300)	18.167 (6.052)	7.833 (2.365)	25.667 (7.415)
12 years (n=35)	19.114 (7.467)	13.886 (6.777)	17.600 (6.269)	12.457 (3.109)	63.057 (20.618)	21.857 (6.367)	11.486 (2.174)	33.343 (7.666)
F	17.736	22.938	37.872	41.516	39.214	12.500	25.422	18.913
P	<0.01	<0.01	<0.01	<0.01	<0.01	<0.01	<0.01	<0.01

Table 4.11 : Mean, Standard Deviation (in parentheses) of Components of Verbal and Non-verbal Creativity Scores of Boys and Girls in a Sample of Children and t-Values

	COMPONENTS OF CREATIVITY							
	Verbal					*Non-verbal*		
	Fluency	*Flexibility*	*Originality*	*Elaboration*	*Total Score*	*Elaboration*	*Originality*	*Total Score*
TRIBAL (n=100)								
Boys (n=52)	14.461 (7.092)	9.827 (5.223)	9.750 (6.277)	7.961 (4.994)	42.000 (21.134)	20.288 (8.419)	10.404 (3.664)	30.692 (11.057)
Girls (n=48)	8.167 (3.527)	5.396 (3.085)	7.187 (3.955)	6.791 (3.326)	27.520 (11.596)	16.464 (7.111)	8.479 (3.389)	25.125 (9.036)
t	5.547	5.110	2.419	1.367	4.198	2.327	2.720	2.744
P	<0.01	<0.01	<0.05	NS	<0.01	<0.05	<0.01	<0.01
NON-TRIBAL (n=100)								
Boys (n=52)	16.326 (7.587)	11.019 (6.731)	13.115 (6.816)	9.327 (3.979)	49.788 (22.602)	19.558 (7.807)	10.019 (2.552)	29.385 (9.629)
Girls (n=48)	12.333 (5.187)	7.687 (4.033)	10.687 (5.520)	8.354 (3.954)	39.083 (15.968)	16.625 (5.437)	8.333 (2.956)	24.979 (7.171)
t	5.187	4.033	5.520	3.954	15.968	2.163	3.058	2.578
P	<0.01	<0.01	<0.01	<0.01	<0.01	<0.05	<0.01	<0.05

In tribal group, the mean score of the total components of non-verbal creativity for boys is 30.692 and for girls 25.125. In the non-tribal group, the mean score is 29.385 for boys and 24.979 for girls.

On the whole t-values indicates the statically significant difference with respect to boys and girls in all verbal except elaboration component and non-verbal components of creativity in tribal children. In the non-tribal group, significant differences are seen with regard to boys and girls in all verbal and non-verbal components of creativity.

From these findings, it is interesting to note that the boys are superior to girls in all components of verbal and non-verbal creativity in tribal and non-tribal groups. A similar trend is shown by a few investigator e.g., Torrance (1967). Straus and Straus (1968), Mar I (1971), Raina (1969), Rawat and Agarwal (1977), Tara (1981), Dharmangadan (1981) and Bhaskara (1986). This may be due to greater socio-cultural encouragement for boys to be original and divergent. Boys do better on figural originality and figural elaboration. This may be attributed to the fact that boys are definitely given more opportunities in Indian culture to manipulate and explore things and have more chances to express their ideas through figures.

In the Indian culture the female children's movements are more restricted than those of the male children. Naturally, it limits their environment when compared to that boys who more about in the surroundings more freely and see several things. This may have naturally affected their score on the Unusual Uses Test.

Recent cultural changes in India have not markedly altered the sex-role restrictions on girls.Girls get few opportunities to expess their divergent thoughts, to take decision in domestic affairs and to solve problems. It is a fact that parents take all decisions minor to major for their daughters, restricting the chances to think of thier own.

Hence it is essential that parents give an opportunity to their daughters to communicate and express freely their unique thinking and analysis. Decision making should be encouraged so that, they would learn to think and act independently.

An examination of the Table 4.12 shows that the mean score of field dependence/independence cognitive style in tribal and non-tribal children is 58.433 and 49.876 respectively which shows high significant difference ($P < 0.01$). The mean score of reflection/ impulsivity

Table 4.12 : Mean, Standard Deviation (in parentheses) of Scores of Cognitive Styles in a Sample of Children and t-values

Cognitive Styles	*Sample of Children (N=200)*		*t*	*P*
	Tribal (n=100)	Non-Tribal (n=100)		
Field dependence/ independence	58.433 (24.135)	49.876 (20.243)	2.716	<0.01
Reflection/Impulsivity	0.508 (0.314)	(0.527) (0.389)	0.382	NS

cognitive style in tribal and non-tribal children is 0.508 and 0.527 respectively which indicates that there is no significant difference.

Field dependence/independence cognitive style is mostly seen in tribal children when compared to non-tribal children. The reflection/ impulsivity cognitive style is equally seen in tribal and non-tribal children.

It is evident from Table 4.13 that the mean values of field dependence/independence cognitive style for 10,11 and 12 years tribal children are 79.058, 59.543 and 36.857 respectively. In non-tribal group, the mean scores for the above mentioned are 69,069, 50.481 and 30.164 respectively. The F-value indicates the significant difference in both tribal and non-tribal groups according to age (P < 0.01).

The mean values of reflection/impulsivity cognitive style for 10,11 and 12 years tribal children are 0.446, 0.566 and 0.519 respectively. F-value shows no significant difference. The mean values of reflection/impulsivity cognitive style for 10,11 and 12 years non-tribal children are 0.329, 0.495 and 0.751 respectively F-value shows statistically high significant difference (P < 0.01).

From the examination of the above findings, it is clear that when the children's age increase in tribal and non-tribal groups, the field dependence/independence cognitive style decreases. In the case of reflection/impulsivity cognitive style, the increasing trend is observed when age increases.

Table 4.14 reveals that the mean scores of field dependence/ independence cognitive style in tribal boys and girls are 54.434 and 62.765 respectively. In non-tribal group, the mean scores of boys and girls with regard to field dependence/independence cognitive style are

Table 4.13 : Mean, Standard Deviation (in parentheses) of the Scores of Cognitive Styles of 10, 11 and 12 Years Age Group in a Sample of Children and F-Values

	COGNITIVE STYLES	
	Field Dependence/ Independence	*Reflection/ Impulsivity*
Tribal (n=100)		
Age Groups		
10 years (n=35)	79.058 (22.737)	0.446 (0.319)
11 years (n=30)	59.543 (12.551)	0.566 (0.301)
12 years (n=35)	36.857 (11.249)	0.519 (0.317)
F	57.256	1.215
P	<0.01	NS
Non-Tribal (n=100)		
Age Groups		
10 years (n=35)	69.069 (14.044)	0.329 (0.170)
11 years (n=30)	50.481 (9.789)	0.495 (0.294)
12 years (n=35)	30.164 (11.602)	0.751 (0.495)
F	91.414	12.951
P	<0.01	<0.01

46.239 and 53.816 respectively. The t-values shows statistical less significant ($P < 0.1$) in both tribal and non-tribal groups according to sex.

In the case of reflection/impulsivity cognitive style, the mean scores of tribal boys and girls are 0.483 and 0.535. On the other hand, the mean scores of reflection/impulsivity cognitive style in non-tribal boys and girls are 0.502 and 0.554. There is no significant difference with respect to sex in both tribal and non-tribal groups.

The mean and standard deviation of CPQ factors in tribal and non-tribal children and t-values are furnished in Table 4.15. It shows that the mean values of A (reserved vs Outgoing), B (Less intelligent vs more intelligent F (Sober Vs Happy-go-lucky), H (Shy Vs Venture-

Table 4.14 : Mean, Standard Deviation (in parentheses) of the Scores of Cognitive Styles of Boys and Girls in a Sample of Children and t-Values

	COGNITIVE STYLES	
	Field Dependence/ Independence	*Reflection/ Impulsivity*
Tribal (n=100)		
Boys (n=52)	54.434 (25.313)	0.483 (0.277)
Girls (n=48)	62.765 (22.244)	0.535 (0.350)
t	1.742	0.823
P	<0.01	NS
Non-Tribal (n=100)		
Boys (n=52)	46.239 (19.636)	0.502 (0.409)
Girls (n=48)	53.816 (20.352)	0.554 (0.368)
t	1.894	0.663
P	<0.01	NS

some), I (Tough-minded Vs Tender-minded), N (Forthright Vs Shrewd), O (Placid vs Apprehensive), Q_3 (Undisciplined, self conflict Vs Controlled) and Q_4 (Relaxed Vs Tense) Factors in tribal and non-tribal children are not significantly different. The similar result was observed by Ulahambal's (1984) study. The remaining factors like C (affected by feelings Vs. Emotionally stable), D (Phlegmatic Vs Excitable), E (Humble Vs Assertive), G (Expedient Vs Conscientious) and J (Trusting Vs Suspicious) showed remarkable difference between tribal and non-tribal children.

On examination, from the Table 4.15, it is found that tribal children scored more mean values on A, B, C, E, F, H, I, J, N and Q dimensions of personality than non tribal children. It indicates that tribal children are more outgoing, more intelligent, emotionally stable, assertive, happy-go-lucky, venturesome, tender-minded, suspicious, shrewd and tense when compared to non-tribal children. Tribal children scored low mean values on D, G, O and Q factors as compared to non-tribal children, meaning thereby they are more phlegmatic, expedient, placid, indisciplined and self-conflict.

Table 4.15 : Mean, Standard Deviation (in parentheses) of Childrens' Personality Questionnaire (CPQ) Scores in a Sample of Children and t-Values

CPQ Factors	*Sample of Children (N=200)*		*t*	*P*
	Tribal (n=100)	Non-Tribal (n=100)		
A	6.550 (1.527)	6.470 (1.314)	0.397	NS
B	3.890 (1.325)	3.690 (1.383)	1.044	NS
C	6.230 (1.489)	5.790 (1.402)	2.151	<0.05
D	4.070 (1.225)	4.840 (1.245)	4.409	<0.01
E	3.280 (1.706)	2.150 (1.009)	5.701	<0.01
F	4.840 (1.841)	4.730 (1.734)	0.435	NS
G	6.700 (1.432)	7.100 (1.675)	1.860	<0.01
H	5.850 (1.604)	5.750 (1.209)	0.498	NS
I	6.770 (1.601)	6.450 (1.684)	1.377	NS
J	5.320 (1.705)	4.400 (1.735)	3.782	<0.01
N	3.920 (1.606)	3.580 (1.444)	1.574	NS
O	3.490 (1.567)	3.620 (1.879)	0.531	NS
Q_3	6.890 (2.015)	6.970 (1.672)	0.305	NS
Q_4	4.030 (1.432)	4.010 (1.894)	0.084	NS

The Profile Similarity Coefficient Value (rp) (Cattell, et. al., 1970) was calculated to examine the similarity/dissimilarity of the personality factors of tribal and non-tribals children. The rp thus obtained was 0.65, significant at 0.01 level indicating that the more similarity in their personality.

The diagrammatic representation of personality profile of tribal and non-tribal children also presented in Figure 4.1.

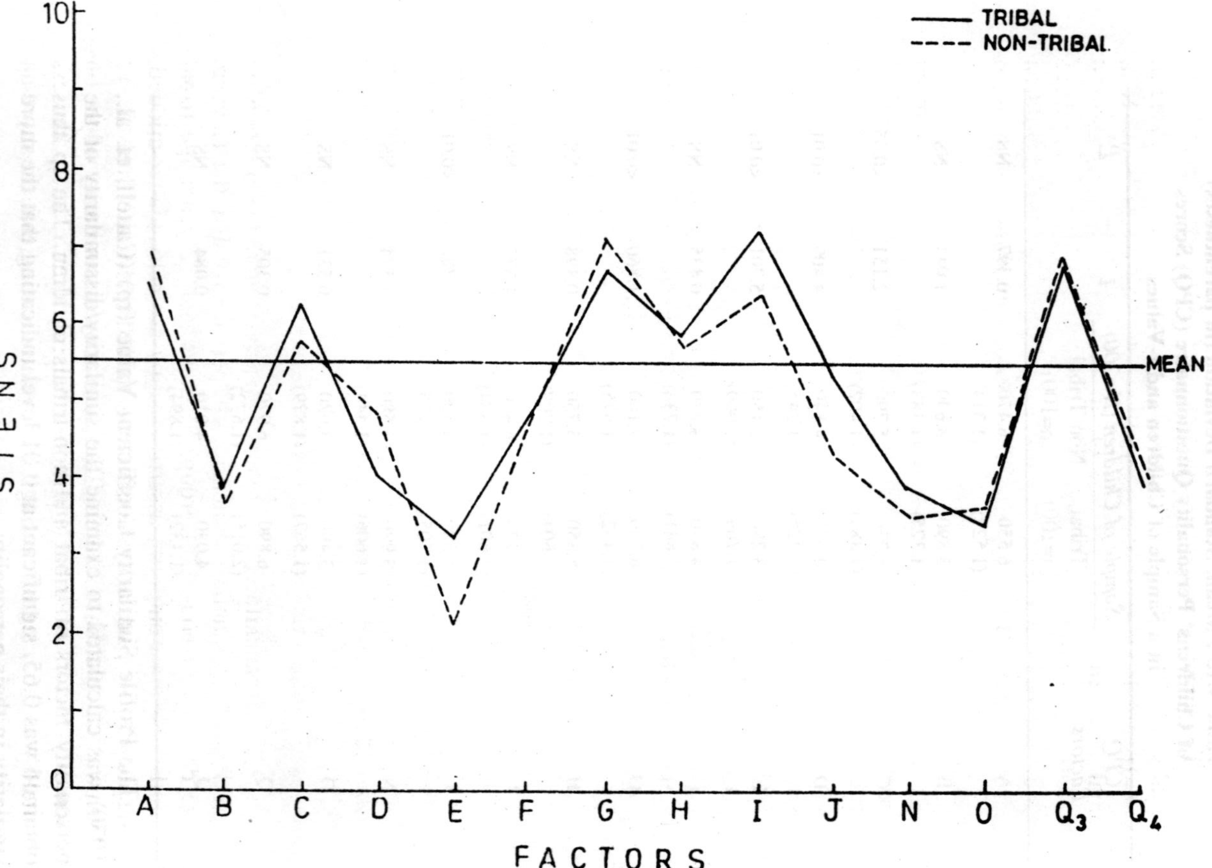

Fig. 4.1 : Personality Profile of Tribal and Non-tribal Children

The mean, standard deviation of CPQ factors in tribal and non-tribal children by age and F-values are given in Table 4.16. (see p. 164–165) It is evident that factors like A,B,C,E,F,G,H,I,J and N in tribal children D,E,G,H,N and Q_3 in non-tribal children showed statistically no significant differences according to age levels (10,11 and 12 years). Remaining factors like D,O, Q_3 and Q_4 in tribal children and A,B,C,F,I,J,O and Q_4 in non-tribal children showed significant differences by age levels.

The Table 4.16 points out that the 10 years age children in tribal group scored higher mean values than the 10 years age in non-tribal children B,C,E,H,I,,J,N, and Q_3. It indicates that tribal children of 10 years age are more intelligent, emotionally stable, assertive, venturesome, tender-minded, suspicious, shrewd and controlled than non-tribal children of 10 years age. They also scored low mean scores on A,D,F,G, O and Q_4 when compared to non-tribal children of the same age, meaning thereby that 10 years tribal children are more reserved, phlegmatic, sober, expedient, placid and relaxed than the 10 years non-tribal children.

The 11 years age tribal children scored more on A,B,C,E,F,G,H and N dimensions of personality that 11 years age non-tribal children which shows that tribal children of 11 years age have more personality traits as outgoing, more intelligent, emotionally stable, assertive, happy-go-lucky, conscientious, venturesome and shrewd than the non-tribal children of similar age group. Tribal children in this age level also scored lower mean scores on D, I,J,O,Q_3 and Q_4 than the non-tribal children meaning thereby that 11 years tribal children are more phlegmatic tough-minded, trusting, placid, indisciplined, self-conflict and relaxed than the 11 years non-tribal children.

The tribal children of 12 years age scored more mean scores on A,E,F,I,J,N,O,Q_3 and Q_4 dimensions of personality than the 12 years age children in non-tribal group. It shows that 12 years age tribal children are more outgoing, assertive, happy-go-lucky, tender-minded, suspicious, shrewd, apprehensive, controlled and tense than the 12 years age non-tribal children. They also scored low mean values on some factors like B,C,D,G and H, meaning thereby they are less intelligent, affected by feelings, phlegmatic, expedient and shy than the similar age group non-tribal children.

The rp value was calculated to observe the similarity/dissimilar-

Table 4.16 : Mean, Standard Deviation (in parentheses) of ∟PQ Factor Scores in Tribal and Non-tribal Children by Age and F-Values

CPQ Factors	Tribal (n=100) Age Level 10 yr. (n=35)	11 yr. (n=30)	12 yr. (n=35)	F	P	Non-tribal (n=100) Age Level 10 yr. (n=35)	11 yr. (n=30)	12 yr. (n=35)	F	P
A	6.086 (1.422)	6.667 (1.516)	6.914 (1.560)	2.801	NS	6.971 (1.294)	6.000 (1.485)	6.371 (1.002)	4.929	<0.05
B	3.743 (1.291)	4.367 (1.066)	3.629 (1.477)	2.951	NS	3.229 (1.477)	3.667 (1.398)	4.171 (1.124)	4.348	<0.05
C	6.229 (1.395)	6.300 (1.236)	6.171 (1.790)	0.059	NS	4.914 (1.292)	5.867 (0.937)	6.600 (1.355)	16.763	<0.01
D	3.314 (1.278)	4.500 (1.009)	4.457 (0.980)	12.681	<0.01	4.743 (1.291)	5.167 (1.416)	4.657 (0.998)	1.533	NS
E	3.686 (1.875)	3.367 (1.691)	2.800 (1.451)	2.486	NS	1.829 (0.747)	2.400 (1.003)	2.257 (1.172)	3.013	NS
F	4.629 (1.664)	5.164) (1.289)	4.771 (2.352)	0.724	NS	5.943 (1.552)	4.200 (1.689)	3.971 (1.248)	17.838	<0.01
G	6.429 (1.461)	7.167 (1.440)	6.571 (1.334)	2.431	NS	7.143 (1.396)	6.767 (1.906)	7.371 (1.716)	1.065	NS
H	6.200 (1.491)	5.600 (1.653)	5.714 (1.655)	1.332	NS	5.629 (1.215)	5.433 (1.455)	6.143 (0.845)	3.187	NS

(contd.)

Table 4.16 : Contd.

CPQ Factors	*Tribal (n=100)* Age Level 10 yr. (n=35)	11 yr. (n=30)	12 yr. (n=35)	F	P	*Non-tribal (n=100)* Age Level 10 yr. (n=35)	11 yr. (n=30)	12 yr. (n=35)	F	P
I	6.486 (1.502)	6.800 (1.540)	7.029 (1.740)	1.014	NS	5.571 (1.420)	6.867 (1.756)	6.971 (1.545)	8.470	<0.01
J	5.514 (1.771)	4.900 (1.668)	5.486 (1.652)	1.311	NS	3.857 (1.717)	5.233 (1.270)	4.229 (1.864)	5.871	<0.05
N	4.429 (1.803)	3.567 (1.591)	3.714 (1.296)	2.873	NS	3.971 (1.504)	3.533 (1.456)	3.229 (1.308)	2.405	NS
O	4.257 (1.657)	3.067 (1.285)	3.086 (1.442)	7.275	<0.01	5.000 (1.831)	3.600 (1.329)	2.257 (1.245)	29.310	<0.01
Q_3	7.543 (1.633)	5.667 (2.412)	7.286 (1.506)	9.411	<0.01	7.257 (1.738)	6.367 (1.519)	7.200 (1.641)	2.907	NS
Q_4	4.571 (1.145)	3.467 (1.196)	3.971 (1.689)	5.274	<0.05	4.800 (1.875)	4.767 (1.524)	2.571 (1.289)	22.195	<0.01

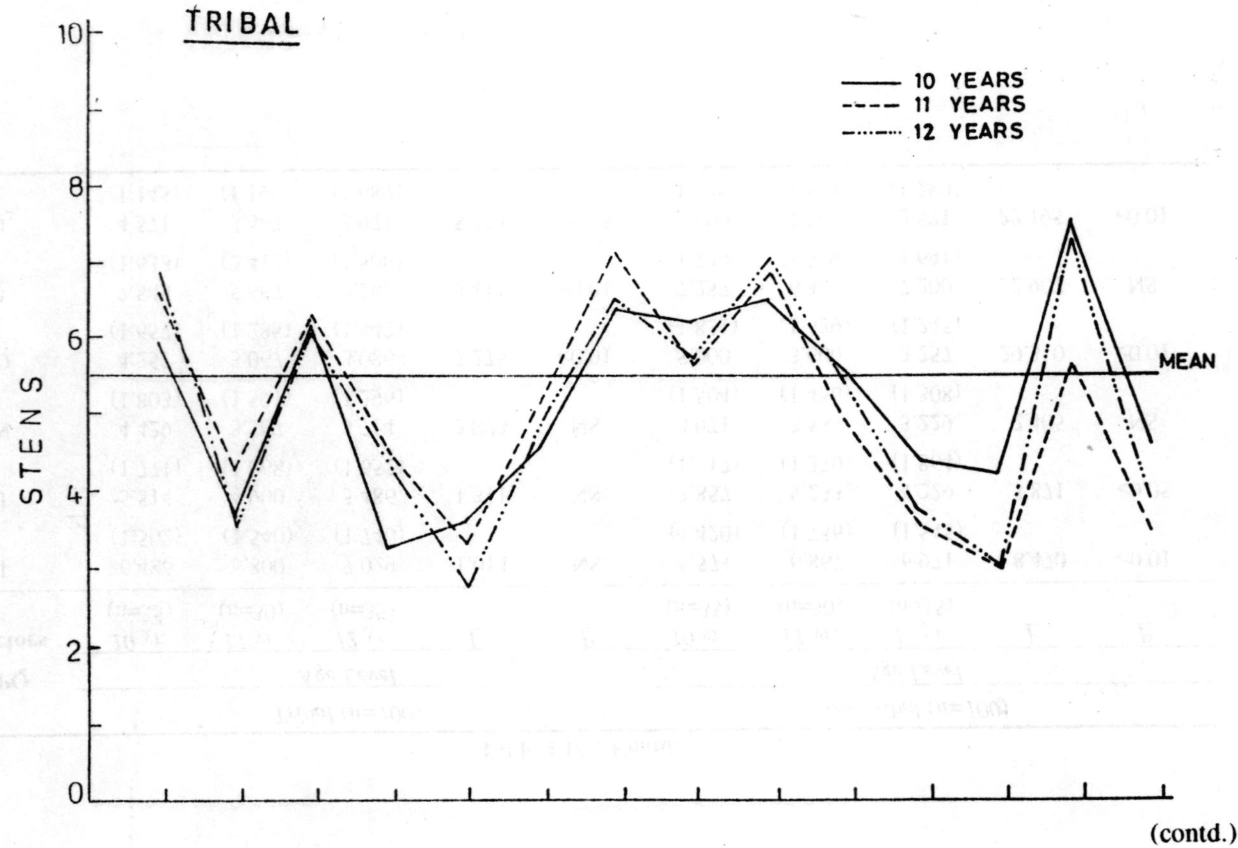

(contd.)

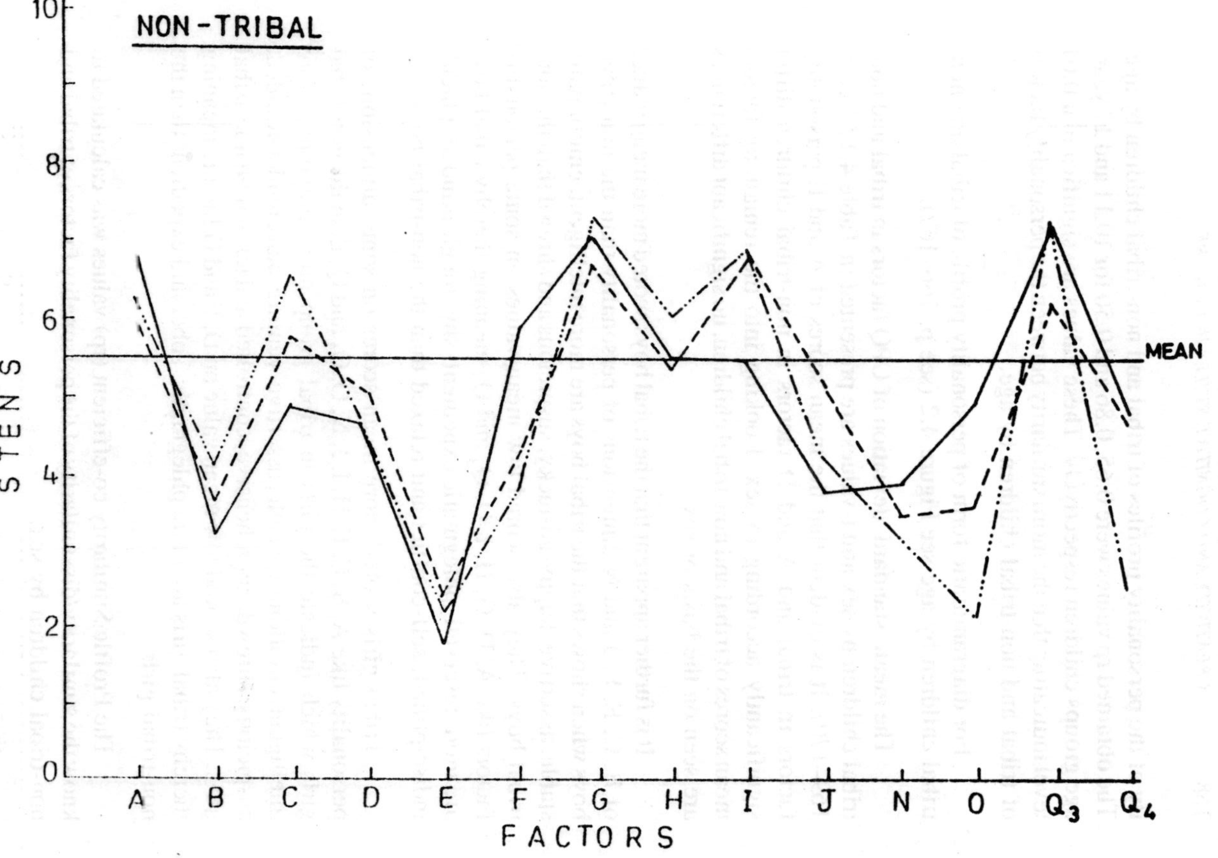

Figure 4.2 : Personality Profile of Tribal and Non-tribal Children by Age

ity of the personality profiles of tribal and non-tribal children by age. The obtained rp values were 0.65, 0.86 and 0.50 for 10,11 and 12 years age groups children respectively. These values are significant at 0.01 level indicating that the more similarity between the personality factors of tribal and non-tribal children by age.

For diagrammatic form of personality profile of tribal and non-tribal children by age see Figure 4.2 (see p. 166–167).

The mean, standard deviation of CPQ factors in tribal and non-tribal children by sex and t-values are presented in Table 4.17 (see p. 169–170). It is evident that the mean scores of A and E personality factors in tribal and A and D factors in non-tribal children differ significantly according to sex. Looking into the remaining factors mean scores of tribal and non-tribal children, no significant differences are seen on the basis of sex.

It is further apparent that the tribal boys scored more mean values of B, C, E, F, J and N dimensions of personality than the non-tribal boys when shows that the tribal boys are more intelligent, emotionally stable, assertive, happy-go-lucky, suspicious and shrewd than the non-tribal boys. They also scored low mean values on some personality factors like A, D, G, H, I, O, Q_3 and Q_4 meaning thereby tribal boys are more reserved, phlegmatic expedient, shy, tough-minded, placid, indisciplined, self-conflict and relaxed than the non-tribal boys.

Tribal girls scored more mean scores on some dimensions of personality like A, B, C, E, H, I, J, N, O, Q_3 and Q_4 than the non-tribal girls which indicate the girls in tribal group more outgoing, more intelligent, emotionally stable, assertive, venturesome, tender-minded, suspicious, shrewd, apprehensive, controlled and tense than non-tribal girls. They also scored low mean value on D, F and G factors meaning thereby tribal girls are more phlegmatic, sober and expedient than the non-tribal girls.

The Profile Similarity co-efficient (rp) values was calculated to know the similarity/dissimilarity of the personality factors of tribal and non-tribal children by sex.

The obtained rp values were 0.84 and 0.49 for boys and girls respectively. These values are significant at 0.01 level indicating that the two groups of children have similar personality pattern by sex.

Table 4.17 : Mean, Standard Deviation (in parentheses) of CPQ Factor Scores in Tribal and Non-tribal Children by Sex and t-Values

CPQ Factors	Tribal (n=100)				Non-tribal (n=100)			
	Boys (n=52)	*Girls* (n=48)	*t*	*P*	*Boys* (n=52)	*Girls* (n=48)	*t*	*P*
A	6.846 (1.601)	6.229 (1.387)	2.051	<0.05	6.865 (1.121)	6.042 (1.383)	3.283	<0.01
B	3.769 (1.198)	4.021 (1.451)	0.948	NS	3.431 (1.393)	3.917 (1.350)	1.586	NS
C	6.385 (1.430)	6.062 (1.549)	1.081	NS	5.885 (1.395)	5.687 (1.417)	0.701	NS
D	4.019 (1.093)	4.125 (1.362)	0.429	NS	5.058 (1.274)	4.604 (1.180)	1.842	<0.1
E	3.654 (1.644)	2.875 (1.696)	2.331	<0.05	2.173 (0.964)	2.125 (1.064)	0.237	NS
F	4.731 (1.783)	4.958 (1.912)	0.616	NS	4.500 (1.935)	4.979 (1.466)	1.387	NS
G	6.827 (1.581)	6.562 (1.253)	0.922	NS	7.269 (1.838)	6.937 (1.479)	0.989	NS
H	5.865 (1.609)	5.833 (1.615)	0.099	NS	5.885 (1.198)	5.604 (1.216)	1.161	NS

(contd.)

Table 4.17 : Contd.

CPQ	Tribal (n=100)				Non-tribal (n=100)			
Factors	*Boys* (n=52)	*Girls* (n=48)	*t*	*P*	*Boys* (n=52)	*Girls* (n=48)	*t*	*P*
I	6.211 (1.446)	7.375 (1.552)	3.880	NS	6.288 (1.741)	6.625 (1.619)	0.998	NS
J	5.461 (1.776)	5.167 (1.629)	0.863	NS	4.596 (1.659)	4.187 (1.806)	1.179	NS
N	3.865 (1.572)	3.979 (1.657)	0.352	NS	3.711 (1.419)	3.437 (1.472)	0.948	NS
O	3.481 (1.788)	3.500 (1.305)	0.061	NS	3.750 (1.898)	3.479 (1.868)	0.718	NS
Q_3	6.654 (2.028)	7.146 (1.989)	1.233	NS	6.885 (1.722)	7.062 (1.629)	0.529	NS
Q_4	3.769 (1.490)	4.312 (1.323)	1.921	NS	4.173 (1.897)	3.883 (1.894)	0.895	NS

The diagrammatic presentation of the personality profile of tribal and non-tribal children by sex is given in Figure 4.3.

From the data presented in Table 4.18 it may be noticed that there

Table 4.18 : Mean, Standard Deviation (in parentheses) of Locus of Control (I–E) Scores in a Sample of Children at t-Values

Locus of Control	*Sample of Children (N=200)*		*t*	*P*
	Tribal (n=100)	Non-Tribal (n=100)		
(I–E) Score	10.230 (1.836)	10.570 (2.138)	1.206	NS

Note : (I–E)—'I' indicates Internal and 'E' indicates External.

is no significant difference with regard to locus of control (I-E) scores between tribal (10.23) and non-tribal (10.57) children.

From the Table 4.19 it may be seen that there is no significant difference with regard to locus of control (I-E) score between tribal and non-tribal children on the basis of age level i.e., 10, 11 and 12 years.

Table 4.20 clearly illustrates that the mean value of locus of control (I-E) scores in tribal boys (10.019) and girls (10.458) is not significantly different. On the other hand in the non-tribal group also, the locus of control (I-E) score in boys (10.615) and girls (10.521) showed no significant differences.

It is apparent from Table 4.21 that the mean scores of HEI factors like B (Control), C (Conformity), (Rejection), F (Punishment), AV (Availability), OP (Opportunity and UT (Utilization) between tribal and non-tribal children are significantly different at 0.05 and 0.01 level of confidence. Other factors like A (permissiveness), E (Reward), G (Protectiveness), H (Nurturance), I (Deprivation of privileges) and J (Cognitive situation) are not significantly different between tribal and non-tribal children.

The mean values of B,C,D,F and G, HEI factors are high in tribal group as compared to the non-tribal group. This shows that the tribal children rarely receive punishment for undesirable behaviour, flexible, realistic moral standards and meets with approval, receive maximum support from parents to strengthen desired behaviour. more opportunities to understand things and situations and act according to his desires and adequate concern about child's needs than the non-tribal children. Punetha's (1980) study also revealed that on the whole tribal

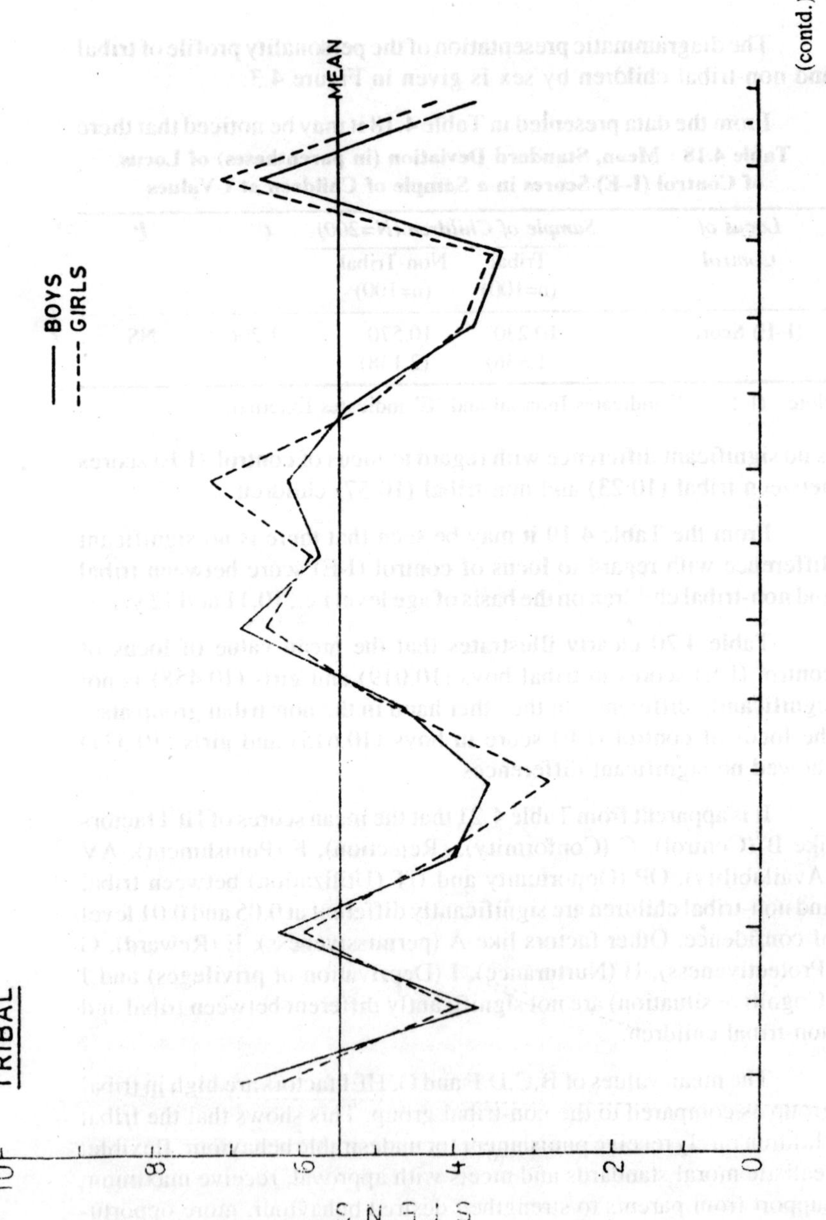

TRIBAL
BOYS
GIRLS
MEAN
STEN
10
8
6
4
2
0
(contd.)

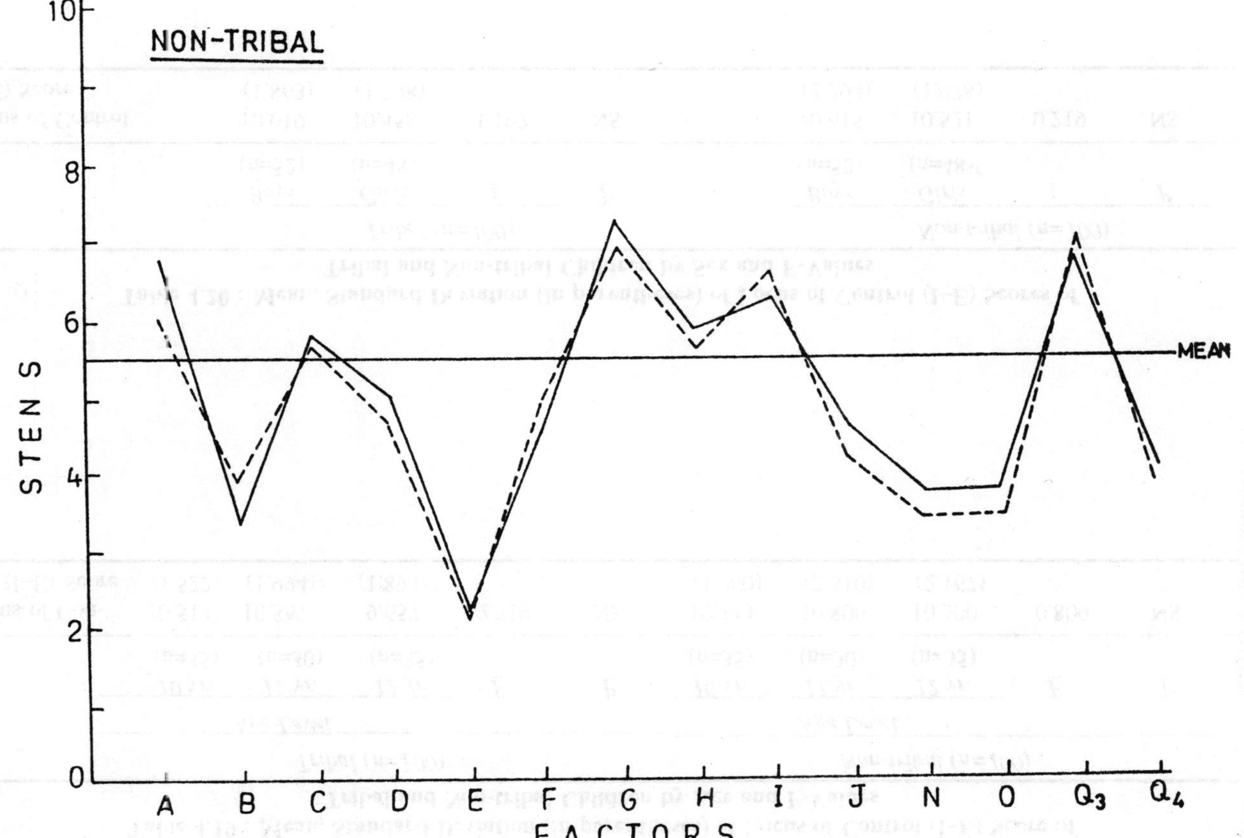

Fig. 4.3 : Personality Profile of Tribal and Non-tribal Children by Sex

Table 4.19 : Mean, Standard Deviation (in parentheses) of Locus of Control (I–E) Score of Tribal and Non-tribal Children by Age and F-Values

	Tribal (n=100)					*Non-tribal (n=100)*				
	Age Level					*Age Level*				
	10 yr. (n=35)	*11 yr.* (n=30)	*12 yr.* (n=35)	*F*	*P*	*10 yr.* (n=35)	*11 yr.* (n=30)	*12 yr.* (n=35)	*F*	*P*
Locus of Control (I–E) Score	10.514 (1.522)	10.567 (1.994)	9.657 (1.893)	2.719	NS	10.743 (1.960)	10.800 (2.310)	10.200 (2.167)	0.809	NS

Table 4.20 : Mean, Standard Deviation (in parentheses) of Locus of Control (I–E) Scores of Tribal and Non-tribal Children by Sex and F-Values

	Tribal (n=100)				*Non-tribal (n=100)*			
	Boys (n=52)	*Girls* (n=48)	*t*	*P*	*Boys* (n=52)	*Girls* (n=48)	*t*	*P*
Locus of Control (I–E) Score	10.019 (1.863)	10.458 (1.798)	1.197	NS	10.615 (2.294)	10.521 (1.978)	0.219	NS

Table 4.21 : Mean, Standard Deviation (in parentheses) of Home Environment Inventory (HEI) Scores in a Sample of Children and at t-Values

HEI Factors	*Sample of Children (N=200)* Tribal (n=100)	Non-Tribal (n=100)	*t*	*P*
A	14.480 (1.967)	14.790 (1.526)	1.245	NS
B	5.100 (1.291)	4.120 (1.113)	5.750	<0.01
C	20.710 (2.969)	19.940 (2.365)	2.029	<0.05
D	16.080 (1.884)	15.540 (1.946)	1.994	<0.05
E	14.560 (1.903)	14.560 (2.114)	0.000	NS
F	14.590 (2.211)	13.660 (2.147)	3.017	<0.01
G	8.380 (1.482)	8.160 (1.354)	1.095	NS
H	9.270 (1.890)	9.510 (1.703)	0.943	NS
I	18.410 (2.625)	18.480 (2.966)	0.177	NS
J	13.710 (2.413)	13.710 (2.687)	0.000	NS
AV	6.220 (2.505)	5.110 (1.847)	3.566	<0.01
OP	6.870 (1.957)	5.760 (1.934)	4.034	<0.01
Ut	6.420 (2.026)	5.520 (2.451)	2.829	<0.01

mothers use more positive forms in handling children's aggressive activities than non-tribal mothers. The positive incentives used are like a material reward, encouraging child verbally in giving up aggressive activities. Tribal children also scored lower mean than the other counterparts on A,H and I HEI factors which indicate that they are highly restrictive, hostile and cold, demands more to work according to parent's desires, insufficient love and attention, limited range of parent guided experience, limited freedom to explore, to experiment and to be independent. Similar mean scores are observed by both tribal and non-tribal group on E and J factors.

With regard to availability (Av), opportunity (Op) and utilization (Ut). The mean scores of tribal group are more than non-tribal group.

On the whole, the total home environment mean score of tribal group is higher than the non-tribal group. It implies the existence of a good home environment in tribal group compared to the non-tribal group.

An analysis of the Table (4.22) reveals that in the tribal group, the mean values of A, B, E, F, H, J and Ut HEI factors and in non-tribal group, the mean values of F, H, J and Av and Op factors differed significantly with respect to their different age levels.

It may be further observed that 10 years tribal children scored more than the non-tribal children of similar age on B, C, D, F, G, I and J factors. This indicates that 10 years age tribal children when compared to the non-tribal children rarely receive punishment for undesirable behaviour, flexible, realistic moral standards, and meet with approval, receive maximum support from parents to strengthen desired behaviour, more opportunities to understand things and situations and act according to his desires adequate concern about child's needs, wide range of parent guided experience, non-freedom to explore, to explore, to experiment and to be independent and lesser exacting disciplinary measures. Tribal children in this age group, also scored lower mean values on A, E and H factors than the non-tribal children meaning there by tribal children have highly restrictive, hostile and cold, prolonged infantile care, unconcern for child's welfare, more individious comparisons and demands more to work according to parents' desires, insufficient love and attention.

With respect to Av, Op and Ut factors, the tribal 10 years age children scored more mean values than non-tribal children of equal age.

The tribal group with 11 years age scored more mean scores than the non-tribal group with 11 years age on A, B, C, E, F, G and H factors. These indicates that tribal children in contrast to the non-tribal children have good home environment like less restrictive, warm and trusting, rarely receive punishment for undesirable behaviour, flexible, realistic

Table 4.22 : Mean, Standard Deviation (in parentheses) of HEI Factor Scores in Tribal and Non-tribal Children by Age and F-Values

HEI Factors	*Tribal (n=100)* Age Level 10 yr. (n=35)	11 yr. (n=30)	12 yr. (n=35)	F	P	*Non-tribal (n=100)* Age Level 10 yr. (n=35)	11 yr. (n=30)	12 yr. (n=35)	F	P
A	13.143 (1.240)	15.733 (2.196)	14.743 (1.521)	20.078	<0.01	14.771 (1.536)	14.400 (1.248)	15.142 (1.683)	1.955	NS
B	5.971 (1.224)	4.733 (0.907)	4.543 (1.197)	16.285	<0.01	4.200 (1.208)	4.067 (0.944)	4.086 (1.172)	0.139	NS
C	20.286 (2.283)	20.733 (3.139)	21.114 (3.419)	0.679	NS	19.857 (2.251)	19.233 (1.869)	20.629 (2.702)	2.957	NS
D	16.400 (1.168)	15.633 (1.732)	16.143 (2.475)	1.378	NS	15.114 (1.659)	15.967 (1.938)	15.600 (2.172)	1.594	NS
E	13.857 (1.192)	14.733 (2.196)	15.114 (2.040)	4.258	<0.05	14.600 (2.145)	14.533 (2.270)	14.543 (2.005)	0.010	NS
F	15.600 (1.265)	14.433 (1.576)	13.714 (2.396)	7.291	<0.01	12.857 (2.415)	14.067 (1.799)	14.114 (1.952)	3.996	<0.05
G	8.800 (1.232)	8.000 (1.576)	8.286 (1.564)	2.538	NS	8.543 (1.421)	7.867 (1.074)	8.029 (1.445)	2.330	NS
H	8.629 (1.437)	9.333 (2.324)	9.857 (1.717)	3.942	<0.05	10.286 (1.934)	9.100 (1.423)	9.086 (1422)	6.173	<0.01

(contd.)

Table 4.22 : Contd.

HEI Factors	Tribal (n=100) Age Level 10 yr. (n=35)	11 yr. (n=30)	12 yr. (n=35)	F	P	Non-tribal (n=100) Age Level 10 yr. (n=35)	11 yr. (n=30)	12 yr. (n=35)	F	P
I	18.514 (2.318)	18.167 (2.913)	18.514 (2.716)	0.181	NS	18.057 (3.638)	19.067 (2.532)	18.400 (2.534)	0.954	NS
J	12.714 (2.094)	14.500 (2.701)	14.029 (2.162)	5.318	<0.05	12.029 (2.361)	15.933 (1.574)	13.486 (2.241)	25.940	<0.01
AV	6.800 (2.459)	5.833 (2.379)	5.971 (2.617)	1.482	NS	5.914 (1.837)	4.267 (1.779)	5.029 (1.599)	7.303	<0.01
Op	7.314 (1.549)	6.700 (2.230)	6.571 (2.047)	1.434	NS	6.600 (1.459)	5.400 (1.545)	5.229 (2.365)	5.624	<0.01
Ut	7.286 (1.619)	5.767 (1.924)	6.114 (2.219)	5.636	<0.05	5.343 (1.644)	5.967 (3.419)	5.314 (2.139)	0.708	NS

moral standards and meet with approval, less interference, more concern for child's welfare, few individious comparisons, more opportunities to understand things and situation and act according to his desires, adequate concern about child's needs and few demands to work according to parent's desires, sufficient love and attention. The tribal children also scored lower mean scores on D, I and J Home Environment Inventory factors than the non-tribal children meaning thereby the tribal children receive minimum support from parents to strengthen desired behavior and too much exacting disciplinary measures, expecting implicit obedience as compared to the non-tribal children.

The tribal children in 11 years age group scored more on Av and Op factors than the non-tribal children. With regard to Ut factor, the non-tribal children scored more than the tribal children.

In the tribal group, the 12 years age group children scored higher mean scores on B, C, D, E, G, H, I and J factors than the non-tribal 12 years age group children. This shows that when compared to non-tribal children, the tribal children rarely receive punishment for undesirable behaviour, flexible, realistic moral standards and meet with approval, receive maximum support from parents to strengthen desired behaviour, less interference, more concern for child's needs, few demands to work according to parent's desires, sufficient love and attention, wide range of parent guided experience, non-freedom on explore, to experiment and to be independent and lesser expecting disciplinary measures. Tribal children also scored lower mean values on some HEI factors like A and F than, non-tribal children which shows that they have highly restrictive, hostile and cold and less opportunities to understand things and situation, more and supervision.

The mean values of Av, Op and Ut factors are more in tribal group with 12 years than in the non-tribal group of same age.

From the Table (4.23), it is clear that only I factor in tribal children and A, G, Op and Ut factors in non-tribal children showed significant differences on the basis of sex.

It may be further seen that tribal boys scored more than the non-tribal boys on B, D, E, F and I HEI factors. This shows that when compared to the non-tribal, the tribal boys rarely receive punishment for undesirable behaviour, receive maximum support from parents to strengthen desired behaviour, less interference, more concern for

Table 4.23 : Mean, Standard Deviation (in parentheses) of HEI Factor Scores in Tribal and Non-tribal Children by Sex and t-Values

HEI Factors	Tribal				Non-tribal			
	Boys	*Girls*	*t*	*P*	*Boys*	*Girls*	*t*	*P*
A	14.635 (2.205)	14.312 (1.678)	0.817	NS	15.077 (1.506)	14.479 (1.502)	1.986	<0.05
B	4.788 (1.288)	5.437 (1.219)	2.582	NS	4.058 (1.145)	4.187 (1.085)	0.581	NS
C	20.173 (3.160)	21.292 (2.657)	1.907	NS	20.211 (2.592)	19.646 (2.078)	1.198	NS
D	16.096 (1.785)	16.062 (2.004)	0.089	NS	15.519 (1.925)	15.562 (1.988)	0.110	NS
E	14.750 (2.085)	14.354 (2.682)	1.039	NS	14.519 (2.296)	14.604 (1.921)	0.199	NS
F	14.923 (2.299)	14.229 (2.076)	1.579	NS	13.654 (2.066)	13.667 (2.253)	0.029	NS
G	8.269 (1.497)	8.500 (1.473)	0.776	NS	8.423 (1.446)	7.875 (1.196)	2.055	<0.05
H	9.288 (2.013)	9.250 (1.768)	0.101	NS	9.788 (1.851)	9.208 (1.487)	1.719	NS

(Contd.)

Table 4.23 : Contd.

HEI Factors	Tribal				Non-tribal			
	Boys	*Girls*	*t*	*P*	*Boys*	*Girls*	*t*	*P*
I	19.038 (2.473)	17.729 (2.639)	2.561	<0.05	18.981 (2.646	17.937 (3.218)	1.776	NS
J	13.788 (2.395)	13.625 (2.454)	0.337	NS	13.904 (2.878)	13.500 (2.475)	0.749	NS
AV	6.038 (2.301)	6.417 (2.719)	0.753	NS	5.269 (1.981)	4.937 (1.694)	0.896	NS
Op	7.058 (2.014)	6.667 (1.894)	0.998	NS	6.500 (1.553)	4.958 (1.999)	4.324	<0.01
Ut	6.365 (1.889)	6.479 (2.183)	0.279	NS	6.615 (2.410)	4.333 (1.894)	5.234	<0.01

child's welfare, few individious comparisons, more opportunities to understand things and situations and act according to his desires and wide range of parent guided experience, non-freedom to explore, to experiment and to be independent.

Tribal boys are compared to the non-tribal boys, also scored low mean values on A, G, H and J measuring thereby they are highly restrictive, hostile and cold, rigid, unrealistic moral standards, meet with disapproval, little concern about child's needs, demands more to work according to parent's desires, insufficient love and attention and too much exacting disciplinary measures, expecting implicit obedience.

With regard to Av and Op factors, tribals boys scored more mean values than the non-tribal boys, But, the means score of Ut factor is more among non-tribal boys when compared to other counterpart.

Tribals girls scored higher scores on B, C, D, F, G, H and J factors than non-tribal girls meaning thereby they rarely receive punishment for undesirable behaviour flexible, realistic moral standards and meet with approval, receive maximum support from parents to strengthen desired behaviour, more opportunities to understand things and situations and act according to his desires, adequate concern about child's needs, fewer demands to works according to Parents desires, sufficient love and attention and lesser exacting disciplinary measures than non-tribal girls. Tribal girls also scored lower mean score on A, E and I factor which shows that they have highly restrictive, hostile and cold, prolonged infantile care, unconcern for child's welfare, more individious comparisons and limited range of parent guided experience, limited freedom to explore, to experiment and to be independent characteristics than non-tribal girls.

The mean scores of Av, Op and Ut are more among tribal girls than among the non-tribal girls.

3. THE RELATIONSHIP BETWEEN CREATIVITY AND COGNITIVE STYLES IN TRIBAL AND NON-TRIBAL CHILDREN

The correlation between creativity (verbal and non-verbal) and cognitive styles (field dependence/independence and reflection/impulsivity) is presented through correlation coefficients in Table 4.24.

In the tribal and non-tribal groups, the verbal and non-verbal

Table 4.24 : Correlation between Creativity (Verbal and Non-Verbal) and Cognitive Styles (Field Dependence/Independence and Reflection/Impulsivity)

Group	*Components of Creativity*	*Cognitive Styles*	
		Field Dependence/ Independence	*Reflection/ Impulsivity*
Tribal	Verbal	-0.391^{**}	0.075^{+}
	Non-verbal	-0.458^{**}	-0.083^{+}
Non-Tribal	Verbal	-0.530^{**}	-0.285^{**}
	Non-verbal	-0.448^{**}	0.146^{+}

Note : $^{**}P<0.01$; $^{+}$Not Significant.

creativity are negatively correlated (P < 0.01) with field dependence/independence cognitive style. That means when creativity score increases, the field dependence/independence score decreases and vice-versa (Interpretation of the score for field dependence/independence indicates higher score for field dependence and lower score for field independence cognitive style). In other words there is significant correlation between creativity and field independence cognitive style. Similar finding was observed by Noppe (1977), Frank and Noble (1985), smilansky and Halberstadt (1986) and Bal (1988) who reported that field independent person is fluent, flexible and original (Torrance's creativity) and also makes remote associations in thinking (Mednick's creativity). Field dependent individual on the other hand is dominated by the overall organisation of the surrounding field and there is less scope of creativity in the cognitive functioning.

In the tribal group, the verbal and non-verbal creativity is not significantly correlated with reflection/impulsivity cognitive style. In the non-tribal group, only verbal creativity is significantly and positively correlated (P < 0.01) with reflection/impulsivity cognitive style. That means when verbal creativity score increases, the reflection/impulsivity score also increases and vice-versa (Interpretation of the scores for reflection/impulsivity indicates higher score for reflection and lower score for impulsivity cognitive style). In other words there is significant correlation between verbal creativity and reflection cognitive style. This result is in line other studies by Kagan and Kogan (1970), Block et al (1974), Fuqua, Bartsch and Phye (1975) and Adejumo (1979).

4. RESULTS OF MULTIPLE (STEP-WISE) REGRESSION ANALYSIS

Multiple (step-wise) Regression analysis was carried to identify the predicators of creativity and cognitive styles. It is understood that several variables either independently or together influence the children's creativity and cognitive styles.

The task of a scientific evaluation involves in establishing how much and how well a set of independent variables having logical bearing on the dependent variable facilitate accurate prediction. This can be accomplished by using Multiple (step-wise) Regression Analysis, a powerful tool developed by statisticians. Hence, the analysis was carried out to identify the various variables which would contribute to creativity and cognitive styles and to develop multiple regression equation which would reasonably predict the dependent variables.

In the present investigation, Multiple (step-wise) Regression analysis was carried out on two dependent variables. Creativity (verbal and non-verbal) and Cognitive Styles (field dependence/independence and reflection impulsivity). Age, Sex, Home Environment and Locus of control (I-E) were treated as independent variables. This analysis was done on tribal and non-tribal groups of children separately.

Creativity (Verbal) of Tribal Children

In this analysis, total verbal creativity scores of tribal children were treated as the dependent variable and age, sex, scores of cognitive style (field dependence. Independence in reflection/impulsivity, total Home Environment Inventory score and locus of control (I-E) score of tribal children were considered independent variables. Multiple (step-wise) Regression analysis was carried out to find out the maximum possible variance in verbal creativity that could be explained with the help of each of the independent variable.

From Table (4.25) it can be seen that in the tribal group, there was no variable entered in the first step. The variable entered in the second step by analysis was age. The multiple correlation (R) was 0.492 which is nothing but zero order correlation between the dependent variable creativity (verbal) and the most influencing independent variable age. The relationship is positive i.e. the higher the age, the higher was the verbal creativity score and the strength of the relationship between the two was about 49.2 per cent. It can also be observed

Table 4.25 : Summary of Multiple (Step-wise) Regression Analysis

Dependent Variable : Creativity (Verbal and Non-verbal). *Independent Variables* : Age, Sex, Cognitive Styles (Field Dependence/Independence and Reflection/Impulsivity) Home Environment and Locus of Control (I–E)

	Step No.	Independent variable entered	Multiple correlation R	R^2	Standard error of estimate	t-value	Partial regression βco-efficient (b)	F-value (degrees of freedom and level of significance	Constant	Zero order correlation with dependent variable and its level of Significance (r)	β-coefficient	Percentage of variance in the dependent variable explained by independent variables
Tribal												
Verbal Creativity	2	Age (1)	0.492	0.242	1.947 (1)	5.597**	+10.900	31.331** (1,98)	13.250	0.492**	0.492	0.242
	3	Sex (2)	0.621	0.386	2.952 (2) 1.763 (1)	4.759** 6.069**	–14.050 +10.699	30.452** (2,97)	34.446	–0.390**).492**	–0.379 0.483	0.148 0.238
Non-verbal Creativity	2	Age (1)	0.524	0.275	1.070 (1)	6.098**	+6.528	37.188** (1,98)	14.963	0.524**	0.524	0.275
	3	Sex (2)	0.582	0.339	1.720 (2) 1.027 (1)	3.086** 6.282**	–5.309 +6.453	24.974 (2,97)	22.971	0.267** 0.524**	–0.255 0.518	0.068 0.271
Non-tribal												
Verbal Creativity	2	Age (1)	0.571	0.326	2.004 (1)	6.884**	+13.800	47.392** (1,98)	17.05	0.571**	0.571	0.326
	3	Sex (2)	0.624	0.389	3.241 (2) 1.919 (1)	3.161** 7.115**	–10.158 +13.655	30.865** (2,97)	32.374	–0.264** 0.571**	–0.251 0.565	0.066 0.323
Non-verbal Creativity	2	Age (1)	0.516	0.266	0.909 (1)	5.961**	+5.386	35.537** (1,98)	16.498	0.516**	0.516	0.266
	3	Sex (2)	0.568	0.323	1.460 (2) 0.872 (1)	2.870** 6.107**	–4.192 +5.326	23.201 (2,97)	22.823	–0.252* 0.516**	–0.239 0.510	0.060 0.263

Note : P<0.05; **P < 0.01.

from the Table that 'R' was significant at 0.01 level (F-value = 31.331 for df = 1,98). The coefficient of multiple determination (R) disclosed that about 24.2 per cent of the variable in verbal creativity was accounted for by age alone in the second step. The standard error of estimate was 1.947 and t-value was 5.597, significant at 0.01 level.

The partial regression coefficient (b) was 10.9. This value indicates that creativity (verbal) increased by 10.9 units for every unit increase in age. The partial regression co-efficient was significant at 0.01 level. The constant value that would be considered in the equation at the end of this step, with which the prediction of verbal creativity would be possible was 13.25. The general form of prediction equation may be given as

$$Y = K + a_1 x_1 + a_2 x_2 + a_3 x_3 + \dots\dots\dots\dots\dots\dots a_n x_n$$

Where Y denotes the predicted score of dependent variable. 'K' is the constant. a_1, a_2, a_3 ....an are partial regression coefficients and x_1, x_2, x_3 .... x_n are the obtained values in different independent variables. Thus the equation at the end of the second step would be

Creativity (verbal) = 13.25 + 10.9 Age ....(i)

Sex was entered into the step-wise regression analysis as the second most significant variable. The multiple correlation (R) obtained between creativity (verbal) on one side and the two independent variables viz., age and sex on the other side was 0.621. Thus, the strength of the relationship between the verbal creativity and the two independent variables put together was about 62.1 per cent. The relationship between creativity (verbal) and sex was negative and significant at 0.01 level (F-value = 30.452 for df = 2,97). The two variables put together could explain about 38.6 per cent $\{R^2 = 0.386\}$ of the variance in the dependent variable, verbal creativity. Out of this 23.8 per cent of the variance was explained by age (1) and the remaining 14.8 per cent was accounted for by sex (2) it was evident that by including sex, the contribution of age decreased from 24.2 per cent to 23.8 per cent due to inter-correlation between the two variables. These percentages were obtained by multiplying the partial regression coefficients (b) with the corresponding zero order correlation between the dependent variable and the respective independent variable (Garrett, 1981).

The standard error of estimate was 2.952. The partial regression coefficient disclosed, when both the age and sex were included as predictor variables, that the creativity (verbal) increased by 10.699, and –14.05 units for every unit increase in age and sex respectively. Both the partial regression coefficients were significant. The regression equation to predict creativity with age and sex as predictor variables was:

Creativity (verbal) = 34.446 + 10.699 Age — 14.05 Sex ....(ii)

The remaining independent variables were not entered in the Multiple Regression Analysis. They are scores of cognitive styles (field dependence/independence and reflection/impulsivity), total HEI score and locus of control (I-E) score. They did not contribute anything to verbal creativity of tribal children.

Creativity (Non-Verbal) of Tribal Children

The total non-tribal creativity scores of tribal children were treated as the dependent variable and age, sex, scores of cognitive styles (field dependent/independence and reflection/impulsivity), total Home environment Inventory score and locus of control (I-E) score of tribal children were counted as independent variables. Step-wise Multiple Regression analysis was done to find out the maximum possible variance in non-verbal creativity that could be explained with the help of each of the independent variables.

From Table (4.25) it is evident that in the tribal group, the independent variable entered in the first step was nill. In the second step, age was entered. The multiple correlation (R) was 0.524 which is nothing but the correlation between the dependent variable, creativity (non-verbal) and the most influencing independent variable age. The strength of the relationship between the two was about 52.4 per cent. It may also be seen that 'R' was significant at 0.01 level (F=37.188 for df=1.98). The coefficient of multiple determination (R^2) was 0.275 which revealed that 27.5 per cent of the variance on the creativity (non-verbal) was explained by age alone. The standard error of estimate was 1.070.

The partial regression coefficient was 6.528 which indicates that non-verbal creativity score increased by 6.528 units for every unit increase in age. The t-value for partial regression coefficient was significant at 0.01 level. The constant value considered in the equation at this step was 14.963. Therefore, the equation with which creativity (non-verbal) would be predicted by age as:

Creativity (non-verbal) = 14.963 + 6.528 Age ...(i)

The next variable that was entered into the analysis was sex. The multiple correlation (R) was 0.582 which indicates the correlation between the creativity (non-verbal) and other independent variables, age and sex. The strength of the relationship between the dependent variable and the two independent variable was 58.2 per cent. It is clear from the Table that 'R' was significant at 0.01 level (F-value = 24.974 for df = 2,97). The value of R^2 (0.339) disclosed that the two variables but together could explain about 33.9 per cent of the variance in the dependent variable, creativity (non-verbal). Out of this, 27.1 per cent was accounted for age (1) and the remaining 6.8 per cent was explained by sex (2), by including sex in the analysis, the variance explained by age had come down from 27.5 to 27.1 per cent due to inter-correlation between the two predictor variables. The standard error of estimate was 1.720. The partial regression coefficients disclosed that when both age and sex were included that the non-verbal creativity score would increase by 6.543 and —5.309 units for every unit increase in age and sex respectively. Both the partial regression coefficients were found significant at 0.01 level. The β-coefficients were 0.518 for age and –0.255 for sex. The regression equation to predict creativity (non-verbal) with age and sex as predictor variable is :

Creativity (non-verbal) = 22.971 + 6.453 Age—5 309 Sex ...(ii)

Where 22.971 was the constant to be considered at this step and partial regression coefficients of age and sex were 6.453 and —5.309 respectively. This was the final step. The remaining independent variables were not entered in the analysis.

The zero order correlation between independent variables and dependent variable as well as inter-correlation with independent variables is shown in Table 4.26.

From Table 4.26, it is interesting to note that in the tribal group, among the independent variables, only age factor shows significant negative correlation with field dependent/independence cognitive style ($P < 0.01$) and locus of control ($P < 0.05$). That means when age increases, field dependence/independence cognitive style and locus of control decreases and vice-versa. In other words, age is significantly correlated with field independence (Interpretation of the score shows that low score for field independence). Crandall and Sinkeldam (1964) also found that older age children exhibited more perceptual indepen-

Table 4.26 : Inter-correlations among Independent Variables and their Correlation with Dependent Variable-Creativity (Verbal and Non-verbal) in Tribal Group

	Age	*Sex*	*Field Dependence/Independence*	*Reflection/ Impulsivity*	*Total HEI*	*Locus of Control*	*Creativity*	
							Total Verbal	*Total Non-verbal*
Age	---	–0.024+	–0.735**	0.097+	–0.031+	–0.196*	0.492**	0.524**
Sex		---	0.173+	0.083+	0.053+	0.120+	–0.390**	–0.267**
Field dependence/ independence			---	–0.010+	–0.083+	0.147+	–0.391**	–0.458**
Reflection/Impulsivity				---	0.127+	0.015+	0.075+	–0.083+
Total HEI					---	0.036+	0.109+	0.021+
Locus of Control						---	–0.223*	–0.255**

Note : $^{**}P < 0.01$; $^{*}P < 0.05$; $^{+}$Not significant

dence. Age also significantly correlated with internal locus of control (Interpretation of score shows that score for internal locus of control)

A significant positive correlation was seen between verbal and non-verbal creativity and age variable. This finding was substantiated by Olshin (1965). Pasi (1972), Raina (1970) and Venkata Rami Reddy and Saleema (1988).

A significant negative correlation was observed between verbal and non-verbal creativity and sex, field dependence/independence and locus of control. When creativity score increases, the scores of sex, field dependence/independence, locus of control decreases and vice-versa.

It is interesting to note that creativity is highly correlated with sex i.e. boys are more creative than girls (Torrance, 1967: Straus and Straus, 1968: Mar I, 1971 Raina (1969: Rawath and Agarwal, 1977: Tara, 1981: Dharmangadan, 1981 Bhaskara, 1986). Creativity is significantly correlated with field independence cognitive style. This finding is in line with Noppe (1977), Frank and Noble (1985), Smilansky and Halberstadt (1986) and Bal (1988). Creativity also significantly correlated with internal locus of control Agarwal and Verma (1977) also found the similar finding.

Creativity (Verbal) of Non-Tribal Children

In this, total verbal creativity scores of non-tribal children were treated as the dependence variable and age, sex, scores of cognitive style (Field dependence/independence and reflection/impulsivity) total Home Environment Inventory score and locus of control (I-E) score of non-tribal children as the independent variables. Step-wise Regression Analysis was carried out to find out the maximum possible variance in verbal creativity which could be explained with the help of the independent variables.

From Table 4.25 it can be seen that in the non-tribal group, none of the variables were entered in the first step. In the second step, age was entered with multiple correlation R = 0.571. The value indicated that the strength of the relationship between the two variables was about 57.1 per cent. It can also be observed from the F-value which is significant at 0.01 level (F=47.392 for df = 1,98). This shows that 32.6 per cent of the variance on creativity (verbal) was accounted by age. The standard error of estimate was 2.004 and t-value was 6.884 (P<0.01).

The partial regression coefficient was 13.8 which indicates that verbal creativity score increased by 13.8 units for every unit increase in age. The partial regression coefficient was significant at 0.01 level.

The regression equation at this step with constant 17.05 and with 13.80 partial regression coefficients for the predictor variable would be:

$$\text{Creativity (verbal)} = 17.05 + 13.80 \text{ Age} \qquad ...(1)$$

The variable sex was entered into the analysis in the third step. It was found that 'R' increased from 0.571 to 0.624. This indicates an increase in the strength of the relationship between dependent variable and two independent variables put together from 57.1 per cent to 62.4 per cent which was significant at 0.01 level (F-value=30.865 for 2 and 97 degree of freedom). The per cent of variance in creativity (verbal) explained by these two variables viz., age and sex was 38.9 ($R^2=0.389$) Out of this 32.3 per cent and 6.6 per cent of variance were accounted for by age and sex respectively. By including sex, the variance explained by age had come down from 32.6 per cent to 32.3 per cent due to inter-correlation between the two variables. The standard error or estimate was 3.214 when all these two variable were considered, the partial regression coefficients indicates that the increase in creativity (verbal) was by 13.665 and –10.158 units for every unit increase in age and sex respectively. The partial regression coefficients of these variables were found to be significant. The sign β-coefficients were 0.565 and –0.251 for age and sex respectively. The regression equation at this step with the constant of 32.374 would be:

$$\text{Creativity (verbal)} = 32.374 + 13.655 \text{ Age} — 10.158 \text{ Sex} \quad ..(ii)$$

Hence, the remaining independent variables were not entered in the analysis. This was the final regression equation.

Creativity (Non-verbal) of Non-Tribal Children

The total non-verbal creativity scores of non-tribal children were treated as the dependent variable and age, sex, scores of cognitive styles (field dependence/independence and reflection/impulsivity) total Home environment Inventory score and locus of control (I-E) score of non-tribal children as independent variables. Step-wise Regression analysis was done to know the maximum possible variance in creativity (non-verbal) that could be explained with the help of each independent variable in non-tribal group.

From Table 4.25, it is apparent that in the non-tribal group, none of the independent variables was entered in the first step. Age was entered with multiple correlation (R) 0.516 in the second step. The value indicated that the strength of the relationship between the dependent variable, creativity (non-verbal) and the most influencing variable age was about 51.6 per cent. It can also be observed that 'R' was significant at 0.01 level (F=35.537 for 1 and 98 degrees of freedom). The coefficient of multiple determination R^2 was 0.266 which revealed that 26.6 per cent of variance on the creativity (non-verbal) was explained by age alone. The standard error of estimate of 'R' was 0.909.

The partial regression coefficient was 5.386. The β-coefficient was 0.516. The t-value for partial regression coefficient was significant at 0.01 level. The equation at the end of second step, with which the prediction of creativity (non-verbal) could be possible was:

$$\text{Creativity (non-verbal)} = 16.498 + 5.386\ \text{Age} \qquad \text{...(i)}$$

Where 16.498 was the constant to be considered at this step and 5.286 was the partial regression coefficient of the variable, age.

In the third step, the independent variable entered was sex with multiple correlation (R) = 0.568. 'R' indicates the correlation between the creativity (non-verbal) and other independent variables age and sex. The strength of the relationship between the dependent variable and the two independent variables was 56.8 per cent. It is clear that 'R' was significant at 0.01 level (F-value 23.201 for 2 and 97 degrees of freedom). The value of R^2 (0.323) disclosed that the two variables put together could explain about 32.3 per cent of the variance in the dependent variable, non-verbal creativity. Out of this, 26.3 per cent accounted for by age and the remaining 6.0 per cent explained sex. The standard error of estimate was 1.46. The partial regression coefficient disclosed that when both age and sex were included the creativity (non-verbal) score would increase by 5.326 and -4.192 units for every unit increase in age and sex respectively. Both the partial regression coefficient were found significant. The regression equation to predict creativity (non-verbal) with age and sex as predictor variable was:

$$\text{Creativity (non-verbal)} = 22.823 + 5.326\ \text{Age} - 4.192\ \text{Sex} \qquad \text{...(ii)}$$

Where 22.823 was the constant to be considered at this step. Other independent variables were not entered in this analysis which indicate no influence.

From Table 4.27, it is clear that in the non-tribal group, there is significant negative correlation ($P < 0.01$) between age and field dependence/independence cognitive style. It shows that when age increases the field independence cognitive style is mostly seen. Age also significantly showed positive correlation ($p<0.01$) with reflection/ impulsivity cognitive style. That means when age increases, the reflection cognitive style is mostly seen. Ault (1973), Campbell and Douglas (1972), Fancher (1969), Kagan (1965), Ward (1973) and Salking and Wright (1977) also supported this result.

The variable sex has significant negative correlation ($P<0.01$) with total Home Environment Inventory score.

Field dependence/independence cognitive style is significantly negatively correlated with reflection/impulsivity cognitive style.

A significant positive correlation exists between verbal creativity and age ($P < 0.01$), reflection/impulsivity, cognitive style ($P < 0.01$) and home environment ($P < 0.05$). In other words, verbal creativity has significant relationship with age, reflection cognitive style, and good home environment (Interpretation of home environment inventory score indicates higher score for good home environment).

To substantiate the relationship between verbal creativity and home environment, Saran (1970) concluded that the child's creativity, curiosity, constructiveness and practical competence depend largely upon the presence of proper home environment.

Anderson and Anderson (1965) also reported that creative expression is more frequent in cultures characterized by less authoritarian attitude toward child rearing and social relationship.

A negative significant correlation was found between verbal creativity and sex (boys are more creative than girls) and field dependence/independence cognitive style.

With respect of non-verbal creativity, the significant positive correlation was found with age ($P < 0.01$), significant negative correlation was seen with sex ($P < 0.05$) and field dependence/independence cognitive style ($P < 0.01$).

Table 4.27 : Inter-correlations among Independent Variables and their Correlation with Dependent Variable-Creativity (Verbal and Non-verbal) in Non-Tribal Group

	Age	*Sex*	*Field Dependence/Independence*	*Reflection/ Impulsivity*	*Total HEI*	*Locus of Control*	*Creativity*	
							Total Verbal	*Total Non-verbal*
Age	---	–0.024+	–0.808**	0.456**	0.028+	–0.107+	0.571**	0.516**
Sex		---	0.188+	0.067+	–0.499**	–0.22+	–0.264**	–0.252**
Field dependence/ independence			---	–0.358**	–0.123+	0.029+	–0.530**	–0.448**
Reflection/Impulsivity				---	0.011+	–0.112+	0.285**	0.146+
Total HEI					---	–0.143+	0.229*	0.194
Locus of Control						---	–0.170*	–0.062+

Note : **P < 0.01; *P < 0.05; +Not significant

Cognitive Style (Field Dependence/Independence) of Tribal Children

In this analysis field dependence/independence cognitive style scores of tribal children were treated as the dependent variable and age, sex, creativity (verbal and non-verbal score, total Home environment Inventory score and locus of control (I–E) score of tribal children as independent variables. Multiple (step-wise) Regression analysis was carried out to find out the maximum possible variance in cognitive style (field dependence/independence) that could be explained with the help of each independent variable.

The Table 4.28 shows that none of the independent variable was entered in the first step. Age was entered in the second step with multiple correlation (R) 0.735. Multiple correlation is nothing but zero order correlation between the dependent variable cognitive style (field dependence/independence) and the most influencing independent variable age. The relationship was negative i.e. the higher age score the lower was the cognitive style score and vice-versa and the strength of the relationship between the two was about 73.5 per cent. It may also be observed from the Table that 'R' was significant at 0.01 level (F-value = 15.255 for df = 1.98). The coefficient of multiple determination (R^2) disclosed that about 54.0 per cent of the variance in field dependence/independence cognitive style was accounted for by age alone in this step. The standard error of estimate was 1.965 and t-value was 10.736 ($P < 0.01$).

The partial regression coefficient of β-coefficient was -21.10. This value indicates that cognitive style (field dependence/independence) increase by -21.10 units for every unit increase in age. The partial regression coefficient was significant at 0.01 level. The β-coefficient was -0.735. The constant value that could be considered in the equation at the end of the first step, with which the prediction of dependent variable would be possible was 100.634. The regression equation at the end of second step would be:

Cognitive style (field dependence/independence) =
100.634 — 21.10 Age ...(1)

The next predictor variable entered in the third step was sex. The multiple correlation obtained cognitive style (Field dependence/independence) in tribal children and the two independence variables, viz., age and sex was 0.751. The strength of the relationship between field dependence/independence cognitive style and the two independent

Table 4.28 : Summary of Multiple (Step-wise) Regression Analysis

Dependent Variable : Cognitive styles (Field Dependence/Independence and Reflection/Impulsivity)

Independent Variables : Age, Sex, Creativity (Verbal and non-Verbal), Home Environment and Locus of Control (I–E)

	Step No.	Independent variable entered	Multiple correlation R	R^2	Standard error of estimate	t-value	Partial regression co-efficient (b)	F-value (degrees of freedom and level of significance	Constant	Zero order correlation with dependent variable and its level of Significance (r)	β-coefficient	Percentage of variance in the dependent variable explained by independent variables
Tribal												
Field Dependence/ Independence	2	Age (1)	0.735	0.540	1.965 (1)	10.736**	–21.10	115.255** (1,98)	100.634	–0.735**	–0.735	0.540
Cognitive Style	3	Sex (2)	0.751	0.564	3.221 (2)	2.326*	7.490	62.925**	89.334	0.173@	0.156	0.027
					1.923 (1)	10.916**	–20.993	(2.97)		–0.735**	–0.731	0.537
Reflection/Impulsivity Cognitive Style	--	--	--	--	--	--	--	--	--	--	--	--
Non-tribal												
Field Dependence/ Independence	2	Age (1)	0.808	0.653	1.432 (1)	13.579**	–19.453	184.398** (1,98)	88.782	–0.808**	–0.808	0.653
Cognitive Style	3	Sex (2)	0.825	0.681	2.311 (2)	2.943**	+6.802	103.741**	78.519	0.188@	0.169	0.032
					1.380 (1)	14.026**	–19.356	(2.97)		–0.808**	–0.804	0.649
Reflection/Impulsivity Cognitive Style	2	Age (1)	0.456	0.208	0.041	5.072**	0.211	25.723** (1,98)	0.105	0.456**	0.456	0.208

Note : @ P < 0.01;* P < 0.05; **P < 0.01.

variables put together was about 75.1 per cent. The relationship was significant at 0.01 level (F-value =62.925 for df=2,97). The two variables put together could explain about 56.4 per cent ($R^2 = 0.564$) of the variance in the dependent variable. Out of this 53.7 per cent of the variance was explained by age and the remaining 2.7 per cent was accounted for by sex. It was evident that by including sex, the contribution of age was decreases from 54.0 per cent to 53.7 per cent due to inter-correlation between the two predictor variables. These pecentages were obtained by multiplying the both coefficient with the corresponding simple correlation between the dependent variables and the respective independent variables.

The standard error of estimates was 3.221. The partial regression coefficients disclosed, when age and sex were included as predictor variables, that the field dependence/independence cognitive style would increase by -20.993 and 7.49 units for every unit increase in age and sex respectively. Both the partial regression coefficients were significant. The regression equation to predict dependent variable with age and sex as predictor variables was;

Cognitive style (field dependence/independence) = 89.334
—20.993 Age + 7.490 Sex ...(ii)

where 89.334 was the constant to be considered at this step and —20.993 and 7.490 were the partial regression coefficient of age and sex respectively.

The other independent variables creativity (verbal and non-verbal) score, total HEI score and locus of control (I-E) scores of tribal children were not entered into the Multiple Regression Analysis.

Cognitive Style ((Reflection/Impulsivity) of Tribal Children

When cognitive style (reflection/impulsivity) scores of tribal children were treated as the dependent variable, there was no independent variable entered in the Multiple Regression analysis.

From Table (4.29), It may be noticed that in the tribal group, significant positive correlation (P.<0.01) exists between age and verbal and non-verbal creativity i.e., when age increases, the creativity also increases. Age also significantly and negatively (P<0.05) correlated with locus of control i.e., when age increases, the locus of control score decrease meaning there by they are internals.

Table 4.29 : Inter-correlations among Independent Variables and their Correlation with Dependent Variable-Cognitive Styles (Field Dependence/Independence and Reflection/Impulsivity) in Tribal Group

	Age	*Sex*	*Verbal Creativity*	*Non-verbal Creativity*	*Total HEI*	*Locus of Control*	*Cognitive Styles*	
							Field dependence/Independence	*Reflection/impulsivity*
Age	---	–0.024^{+}	–0.492**	0.524**	–0.031^{+}	–0.196	–7.35**	0.097^{+}
Sex		---	–0.390**	–0.267**	–0.053^{+}	0.120^{+}	0.173^{+}	0.083^{+}
Verbal creativity			---	0.751**	0.109^{+}	–0.223*	–0.391**	0.075^{+}
Non-verbal creativity				---	0.021^{+}	–0.225**	–0.458**	–0.083^{+}
Total HEI					---	0.036	–0.083+	0.127^{+}
Locus of Control						---	0.147+	0.015^{+}

Note : **P < 0.01; *P < 0.05; $^{+}$Not significant

There is highly negative (P<0.01) correlation between sex variable and verbal and non-verbal creativity which indicate that boys are more creative than girls.

Verbal creativity is positively correlated (P<0.01) with non-verbal creativity. Verbal and non-verbal creativity is negatively correlated with locus of control.

Field dependence/independence cognitive style is highly negatively correlated (P>0.01) with age, verbal creativity and non-verbal creativity.

With regard to reflection/ impulsivity cognitive style, no significant correlation was found with any independent variable.

Cognitive Style (Field Dependence/Independence) of Non-tribal Children

In this total field dependence/independence cognitive style scores of non-tribal children were treated as the dependent variable and age, sex creativity score (verbal and non-verbal), total Home environment Inventory Score and locus of control (I-E) score of non-tribal children as independent variables Multiple (step-wise) Regression Analysis was done to find out the maximum possible variance in cognitive style (field dependence/independence) that could be explained with the help of each of the independent variables.

From Table 4.28 it is seen that in the non-tribal group, there was no variable entered in the first step. The important variable 'age' was entered in the second step with multiple correlation (R) 0.808. The strength of the relationship between the two variables was about 80.8 per cent. It is also be observed that 'R' was significant at 0.01 level (F=184.398 for df = 1,98). The coefficient of multiple determination (R^2) disclosed that about 6.53 per cent of the variance in cognitive style (field dependence/independence) was accounted for by age alone. The standard error or estimate was 1.432.

The partial regression coefficient was -19.453 which indicates that cognitive style (field dependence/independence) score increases by -19.453 units for every unit, increases in age, the t-value for partial regression coefficient was significant at 0.01 level. The β-coefficient was -0.808. The equation at the end of this step, with which the prediction of dependent variable would be possible was:

Cognitive style (field dependence/independence) = 88.782
—19.453 Age ...(i)

Where 88.782 was the constant to be considered at this step and –19.453 was the partial regression coefficient of the variable, age.

The next variable entered into the third step of Multiple Regression Analysis was sex. The multiple correlation R was 0.825. The strength of the relationship between the dependent variable and the two independent variables was 82.5 per cent. It is clear from the Table that 'R' was significant at 0.01 level (F value = 103.741 for 2 and 97 degrees of freedom). The value of R^2 (0.681) disclosed that 68.1 per cent of variance on field dependence/independence cognitive style was explained by two variables. The variance contributed by age and sex are 64.9 per cent and 3.2 per cent respectively. It may be noted that by including sex, the contribution of age as brought down from 65.3 to 64.9 per cent due to inter-correlation between the two variables. The standard error of estimate was 2.311. The partial regression coefficient was significant at 0.01 level. The β-coefficient for these two variables were -0.804 (age) and 0.169 (sex). The t-values for age and sex were 14.026 and 2.943 ($P < 0.01$). the prediction equation at this step with the constant 78.519 and the partial regression coefficient, -19.356 for age and 6.802 for sex would be;

Cognitive style (field dependence/independence) = 78.519
—19.356 Age + 6.802 Sex ...(ii)

The other independent variables were not entered into the analysis. This was the final step.

Cognitive Style (Reflection/Impulsivity) of Non-tribal Children

The cognitive style (reflection/impulsivity) scores of non-tribal children were treated as the dependent variable and age, sex, creativity score, (verbal and non-verbal) the total Home Environment Inventory score and locus of control (I-E) score of non-tribal children as the independent variables. Multiple (step-wise) Regression analysis was carried out to find out the maximum possible variance in cognitive style (reflection/impulsivity) that could be entered with the help of the independent variables.

From Table 4.28 it is understood that when the reflection/ impulsivity cognitive style was treated as the dependent variable, only age was entered in the second step. The multiple 'R' was 0.456 which indicates the correlation between the cognitive style (reflection/impulsivity) and the other independent variables like age. The strength of the relationship between the dependent variable and the independent variables was 45.6 per cent. It is clear that the 'R' was significant at 0.01 level (F-value =25.723 for 1 and 98 degrees of freedom). The R^2 disclosed that about 20.8 per cent of the variance in cognitive style (reflection/impulsivity) was accounted for by age alone. The standard error of estimate was 0.041.

The partial regression coefficient was 0.211 which indicates that reflection/impulsivity cognitive style score increases by 0.211 units for every unit increase in age. The t-value for partial regression coefficient was significant at 0.01 level. The equation at the end of this final step, with which the prediction of cognitive style (reflection/impulsivity) would be possible was:

Cognitive style (reflection/impulsivity) = 0.105 + 0.211 Age ...(i)

where 0.105 was the constant to be considered and 0.211 was the partial regression coefficient of the age variable.

The other independent variables were not entered in this analysis. Even sex variable was not entered which means it does not influence the cognitive style (reflection/impulsivity) of the non-tribal children.

Table 4.30 illustrates that in the non-tribal group, the highly significant positive correlation was seen between age and verbal and non-verbal, creativity meaning there by when age increases, creativity also increases.

Negative correlation was found between sex and verbal and non-verbal creativity i.e., boys are more creative than girls. Sex is also negatively correlated with home environment.

Verbal and non-verbal creativity are significantly positively correlated and they both are positively related ($P>0.05$) to home environment.

Field dependence/independence cognitive style has highly significant negative correlation with age verbal and non-verbal creativity.

With reference to reflection/impulsivity cognitive style, there is highly significant positive relationship with age and verbal creativity.

Table 4.30 : Inter-correlations among Independent Variables and their Correlation with Dependent Variable-Cognitive Styles (Field Dependence/Independence and Reflection/Impulsivity) in Non-tribal Group

	Age	*Sex*	*Verbal Creativity*	*Non-verbal Creativity*	*Total HEI*	*Locus of Control*	*Cognitive Styles*	
							Field dependence/Independence	*Reflection/impulsivity*
Age	---	–0.024⁺	–0.571**	0.516**	0.028⁺	–0.107⁺	–0.808**	0.456**
Sex		---	0.0264**	–0.252*	–0.499**	–0.022⁺	0.188⁺	0.067⁺
Verbal creativity			---	0.568**	0.229*	–0.170⁺	–0.520**	0.285**
Non-verbal creativity				---	0.194*	–0.062⁺	–0.448**	0.146⁺
Total HEI					---	–0.143	–0.123⁺	–0.011⁺
Locus of Control						---	0.029⁺	–0.112⁺

Note : **$P < 0.01$; *$P < 0.05$; ⁺Not significant

5. PERSONALITY PROFILES ACCORDING TO DIFFERENT LEVELS OF CREATIVITY AND DIFFERENT COGNITIVE STYLES

Mean values of Children's Personality Questionnaire scores at different levels of verbal creativity in tribal and non-tribal children is given in Table (4.31).

Table 4.31 : Mean Values of Children's Personality Questionnaire Scores at Different Levels of Verbal Creativity in Tribal and Non-tribal Children

	Sample of Children (N=200)					
	Tribal (n=100)			*Non-tribal (n=100)*		
CPQ Factors	High Crea-tives	Average Crea-tives	Low Crea-tives	High Crea-tives	Average Crea-tives	Low Crea-tives
A	6.86	6.4	6.69	7.22	6.44	5.88
B	6.19	6.6	5.79	5.55	7.00	5.57
C	5.43	6.3	5.1	4.51	5.0	4.64
D	5.43	4.7	5.23	6.45	5.44	6.01
E	6.0	5.8	6.44	4.98	5.22	5.0
F	5.48	5.6	4.79	5.0	4.78	4.86
G	6.11	5.2	5.71	5.94	5.67	6.55
H	6.9	6.7	6.31	6.45	5.55	6.28
I	6.69	6.6	5.94	6.24	5.55	5.83
J	7.62	7.6	7.17	5.67	6.55	5.69
N	6.48	5.1	6.31	6.0	5.33	5.64
O	6.5	6.7	6.31	6.53	6.22	6.24
Q_3	6.0	6.8	5.54	6.20	5.55	6.31
Q_4	5.98	6.3	6.48	6.04	6.11	6.76

Figure 4.4 shows that personality profiles of tribals and non-tribal children at high, average and low levels of verbal creativity. An examination of this Figure reveals that in the tribal group, the mean score of high creative children are more than the mean scores of low creative children on A, B, C, D, F, G, H, I, J, N, O and Q_3 dimensions of personality. This indicates that when compared to low creatives,

high creative in tribal group are more outgoing, intelligent, emotionally stable, happy-go-lucky-conscientious, venturesome, tender-minded, suspicious, shrewd, apprehensive and controlled. Some of these results are in consonance with the findings of Barron (1963), Patel (1976), Bhattacharya (1978), Jhag, (1979) Maddu (1980), Kishore (1981), Agarwal and Bohra (1982) and Goyal (1984). High creatives scored low mean values than the low creatives on E and Q dimensions of personality which shows that the high creatives are more humble and relaxed than that of the low creatives.

In the non-tribal group, the mean scores of high creative children are more than the low creative on A, D, F, H, I, N and O dimensions of personality. It indicates that high creatives are more outgoing, excitable, happy-go-lucky, venturesome, tender-minded, shrewd and apprehensive. Some of these findings are supported by Patel (1976), Bhattacharya (1978), Jhag (1979), Kishore (1981) and Agarwal and Bohra (1982).

Equal mean scores were obtained for the high and the low creatives on B, E and J factors. High creatives scored lower mean scores than the low creatives on C, E, G, Q_3 and Q_4 factors which shows that the high creative are more affected by feelings, humble, expedient, indisciplined, self-conflict and relaxed than the low creatives.

The Profile Similarity Coefficient (rp) was computed to examine the similarity/dissimilarity of the personality of tribal and non-tribal high, average and low creative children. In verbal creativity with regard to high creatives the rp value thus obtained was 0.360, significant at 0.05 level, indicating that the high creatives in tribal and non-tribal groups and similar personality profiles. For average creatives, the calculated rp was 0.275, which is not significant. It shows the dissimilarity of personality profiles. In the case of the low creatives, the rp value obtained was 0.6 which is significant t0.01 level indicating that the low creatives in tribal and non-tribal groups have more similar personality profiles.

Mean values of children's Personality Questionnaire scores at different levels of non-verbal creativity in tribal and non-tribal children is given in Table (4.32).

Figure 4.5 indicates that personality profiles of tribal and non-tribal children at different levels of non-verbal creativity like high,

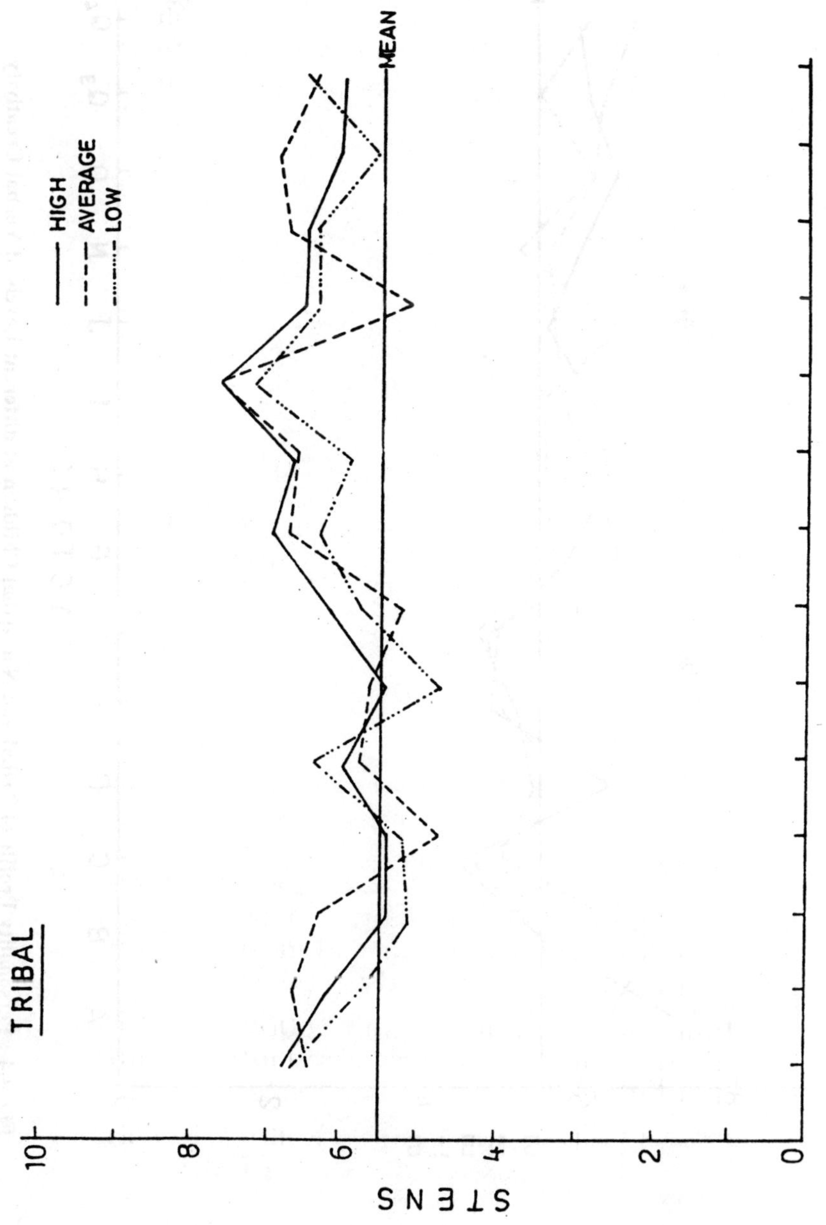
TRIBAL
HIGH
AVERAGE
LOW
MEAN
STENS
10
8
6
4
2
0

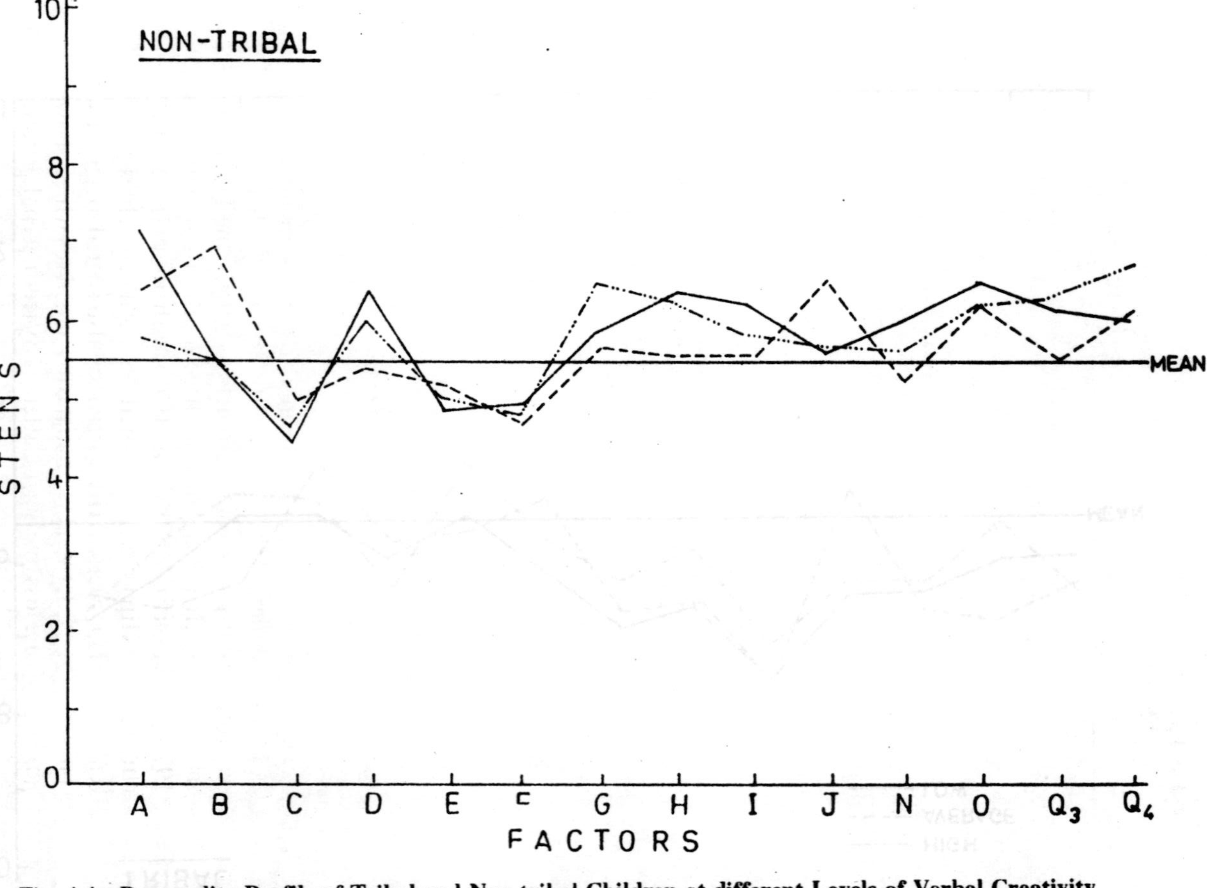

Fig. 4.4 : Personality Profile of Tribal and Non-tribal Children at different Levels of Verbal Creativity

Table 4.32 : Mean Values of Children's Personality Questionnaire Scores at Different Levels of Verbal Creativity in Tribal and Non-tribal Children

CPQ Factors	*Sample of Children (N=200)*					
	Tribal (n=100)			*Non-tribal (n=100)*		
	High Crea-tives	Average Crea-tives	Low Crea-tives	High Crea-tives	Average Crea-tives	Low Crea-tives
A	7.07	6.62	6.76	7.39	4.5	6.19
B	6.07	6.62	6.51	5.86	6.17	5.45
C	5.21	5.5	5.62	4.91	4.33	4.51
D	5.14	6.75	5.58	6.72	6.83	5.76
E	5.93	6.75	6.81	5.14	5.17	4.82
F	5.42	5.62	5.25	5.65	2.93	4.67
G	6.00	5.5	6.04	6.32	7.33	6.09
H	6.90	6.37	6.57	6.44	4.83	6.57
I	6.23	7.0	6.7	6.67	7.5	5.70
J	7.44	6.25	7.63	5.77	5.0	5.86
N	6.65	5.5	6.36	7.11	7.09	5.63
O	6.58	5.75	6.85	6.72	6.33	6.79
Q_3	6.19	5.75	6.15	6.37	5.5	5.86
Q_4	6.39	5.62	6.64	6.12	5.33	6.23

average and low. It is apparent that in the tribal group, the mean scores of high creatives are greater than the mean scores of low creative group on A, F, H and N dimensions of personality. It indicates that the high creatives are more out-going, happy-go-lucky, venturesome and shrewd than that of the low creatives. Some of these results are supported by Patel (1976), Bhattacharya (1978). Jhag (1979), Kishore (1981), Agarwal and Bohra (1982). High creatives scored similar mean values as low creatives on G and Q_3 factors. High creatives also scored lower mean scores on B, C, D, E, I, J, O and Q_3 than the low creatives which shows that high creatives are less intelligent, affected by feelings, phlegmatic, humble, tough-minded, trusting, placid and indisciplined than the low creatives. Maddu (1980) indicated that the high creative group was found to be negatively correlated with intelligence.

In the non-tribal group, the mean scores of high creative children are more than the mean scores of low creative children on A, B, C, D, E, F, G, I, N and Q_3 thereby indicating that the high creatives are more outgoing, intelligent emotionally stable, excitable, assertive, happy-go-lucky, conscientious, tender-minded, shrewd and controlled than the low creatives. Some of these results were substantiated by Barron (1968). Patel (1976), Bhattacharya (1978), Jhag (1979), Maddu (1980), Kishore (1981), Agarwal and Bohra (1982) and Goyal (1984). High creatives obtained lower mean scores than the low creatives on H, J, O and Q_3 dimensions of personality which indicates that the high creatives are more shy, trusting, placid relaxed than the low creatives.

The Profile Similarity Coefficient (rp) value was calculated to examine the similarity/dissimilarity of the personality of tribal and non-tribal high, average and low creative children in non-verbal groups have more similar personality profiles. For the average and low creatives, the obtained rp values were 0.23 and 0.08 which are not significant. It shows the dissimilarity of personality profiles in tribal and non-tribal group.

One the whole, Torrance (1965) reported the selected characteristics of the 'ideal', creative personality in Indian culture are as follows: curiosity, obedience, does work on time, courtesy, health, self-confident, self-starting, industrious, affectionateness, determination. Shainess (1989) stated factors that seem to be important in the creative child with extraordinary potential include (1) good biologic endowment; (2) foestering of interests by parent or interested adult; (3) feelings of being valued and loved; (4) allowance of freedom of development; (5) good toleration of isolation of loneliness; (6) the ability to perceive similarities in the apparently dissimilar; and (7) capacity for love and spirituality.

Mean values of children's Personality Questionnaire scores at field dependence/independence cognitive style is given in Table 4.33.

Personality profile of tribal and non-tribal children at field dependence/independence cognitive style is depicted in Figure 4.6. In tribal group, the field dependents scored higher mean scores on B, E, F, G, J, N and O factors than the field independents. It indicates that the field dependent are more intelligent, assertive, happy-go-lucky conscientious, suspicious, shrewd and apprehensive, than that of the field independents. Field dependents also scored lower mean scores on

Table 4.33 : Mean Values of Children's Personality Questionnaire Scores at Field Dependence/Independence Cognitive Style

	Sample of Children (N=200)					
	Tribal (n=100)			*Non-tribal (n=100)*		
CPQ Factors	Field Depen-dents	Unclas-sified	Field Indepe-ndents	Field Depen-dents	Unclas-sified	Field Indepe-dents
A	6.39	8.0	6.93	6.88	5.5	6.45
B	6.49	6.62	5.63	5.19	5.25	6.11
C	4.9	4.75	5.71	3.71	4.25	6.14
D	5.09	5.37	5.51	5.86	7.75	6.42
E	6.39	5.37	6.36	4.71	5.25	5.14
F	5.18	6.75	4.83	6.69	4.5	3.82
G	5.92	6.37	5.56	6.12	7.5	6.36
H	6.35	6.25	6.71	3.83	7.0	5.8
I	6.11	5.62	6.46	5.57	7.5	6.33
J	7.19	7.12	6.88	5.07	5.5	6.2
N	6.53	6.12	6.05	6.14	5.25	5.56
O	6.84	5.0	6.22	7.14	5.5	6.0
Q_3	5.72	6.75	6.17	6.07	5.75	5.96
Q_4	5.31	5.87	6.12	6.78	7.75	5.36

A, C, D, H, I, Q_3 and Q_4 than the field independents thereby pointing out that they are more reserved affected by feelings, phlegmatic, shy, tough minded, indisciplined, self-conflict and relaxed than the field independents.

In non-tribal group, the field dependents scored more mean values, on A, F, N, O, Q_3 and Q_4 factors than the field independents thereby indicating that the field dependents more outgoing, happy-go-lucky, shrewd, apprehensive, controlled and tense than the field independents. They also scored lower man values on B, C, D, E, G, H, I and J dimensions of personality than the field independents. It shows that field dependents have more personality factors as less intelligently affected by feelings, phlegmatic, humble expedient, shy, tough-minded and trusting than the field independents.

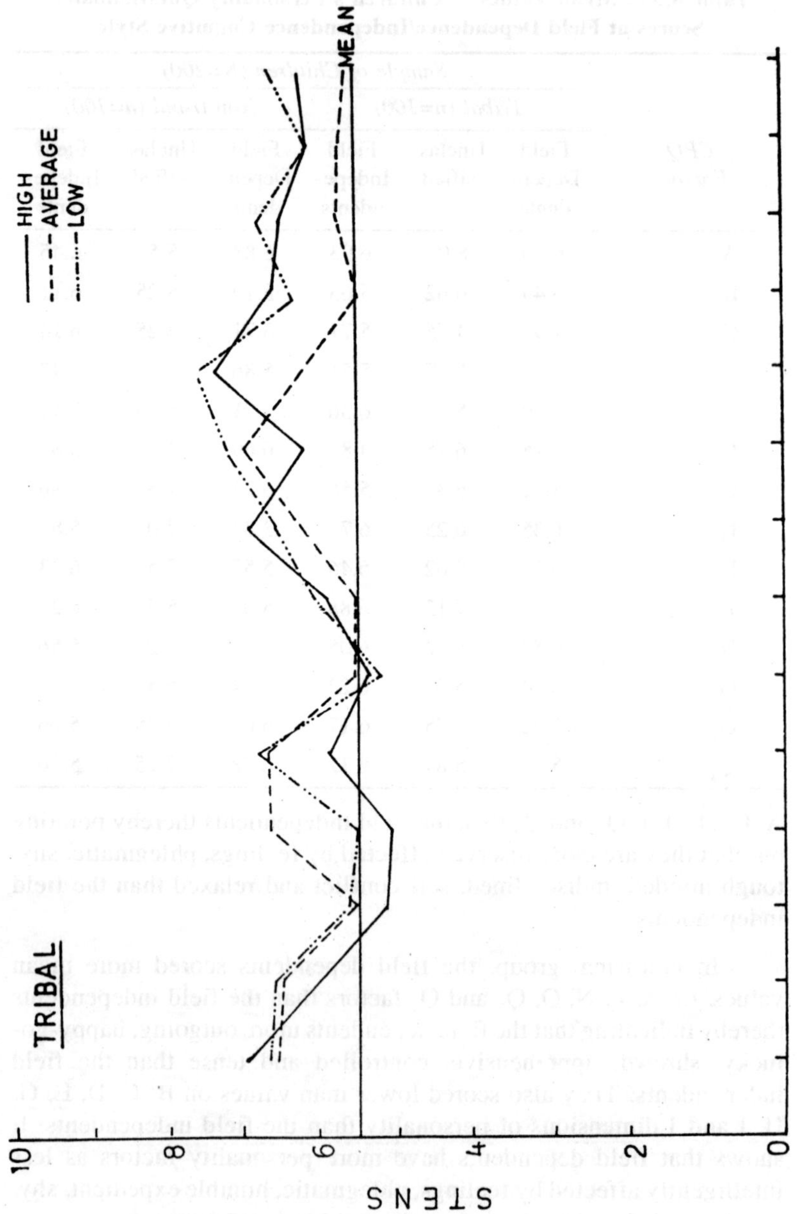
HIGH
AVERAGE
LOW
TRIBAL
MEAN
10
8
6
4
2
0
STENS

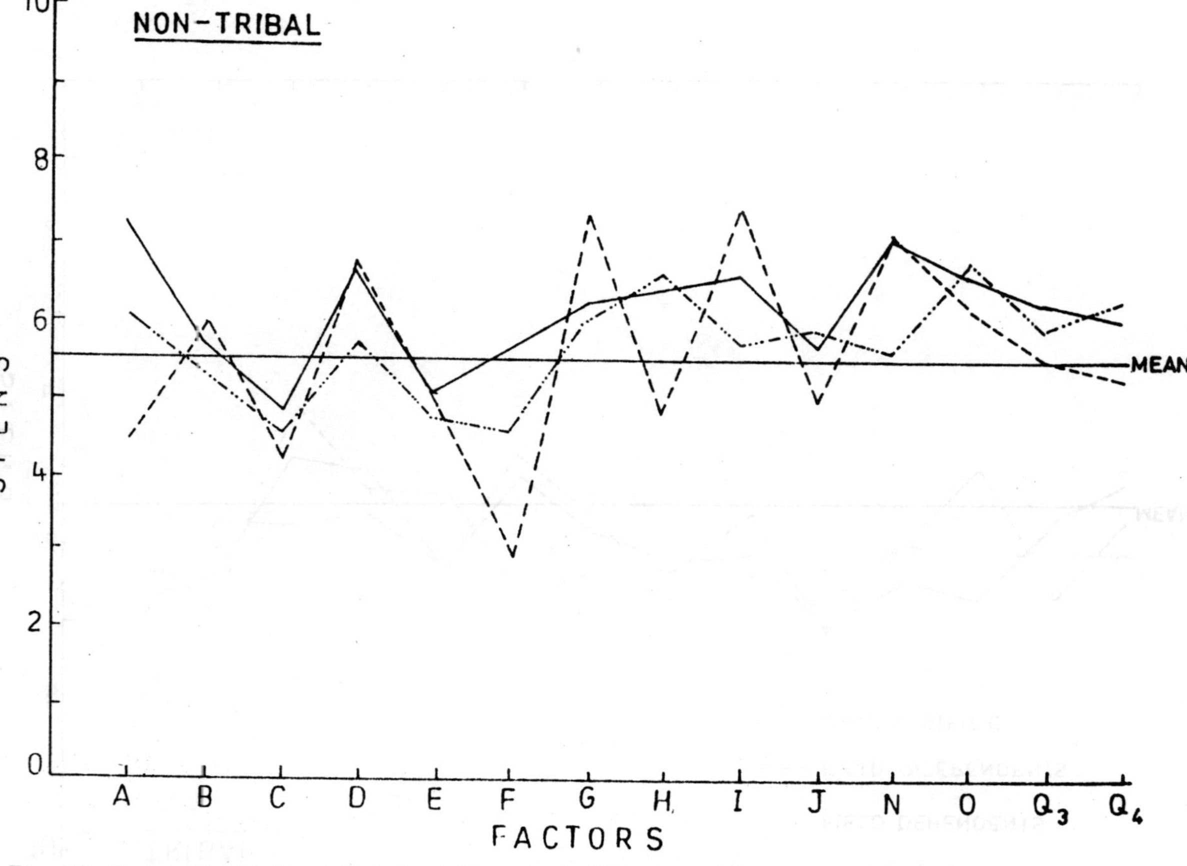

Fig. 4.5 : Personality Profile of Tribal and Non-tribal Children at different Levels of Non-verbal Creativity

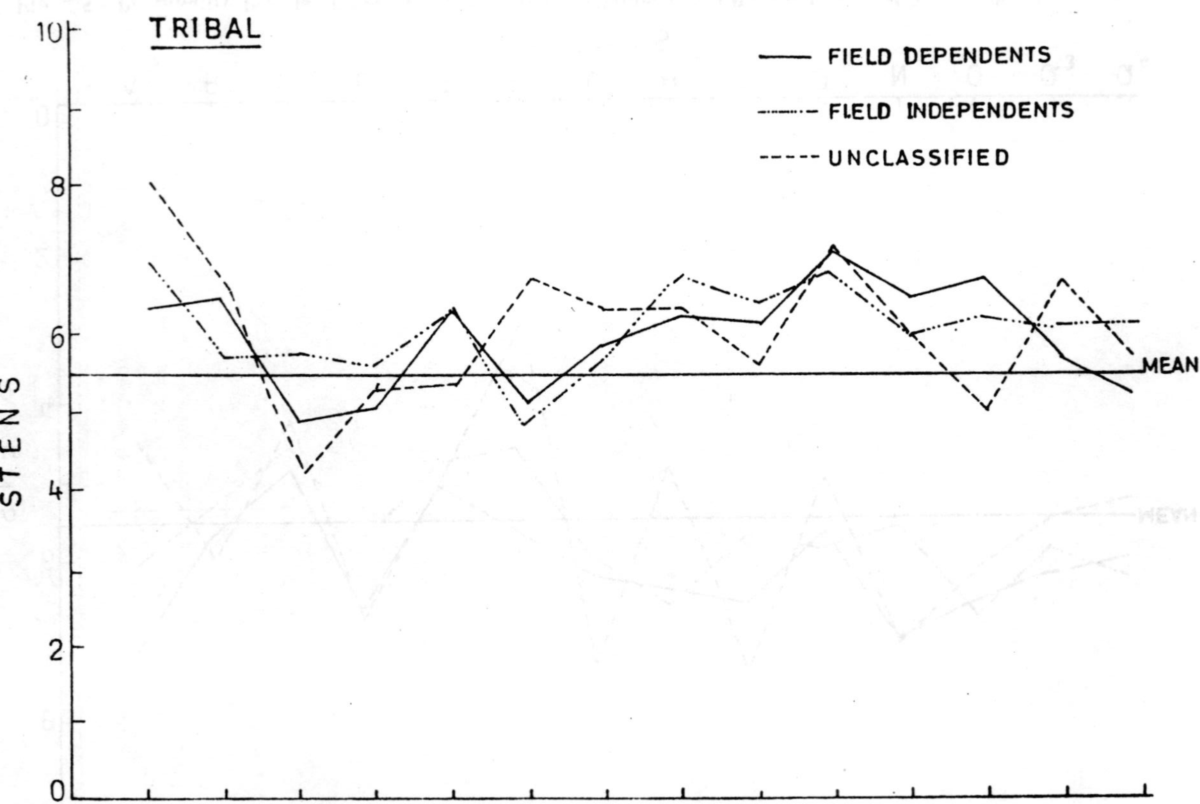
TRIBAL
FIELD DEPENDENTS
FIELD INDEPENDENTS
UNCLASSIFIED
MEAN
STENS
10
8
6
4
2
0

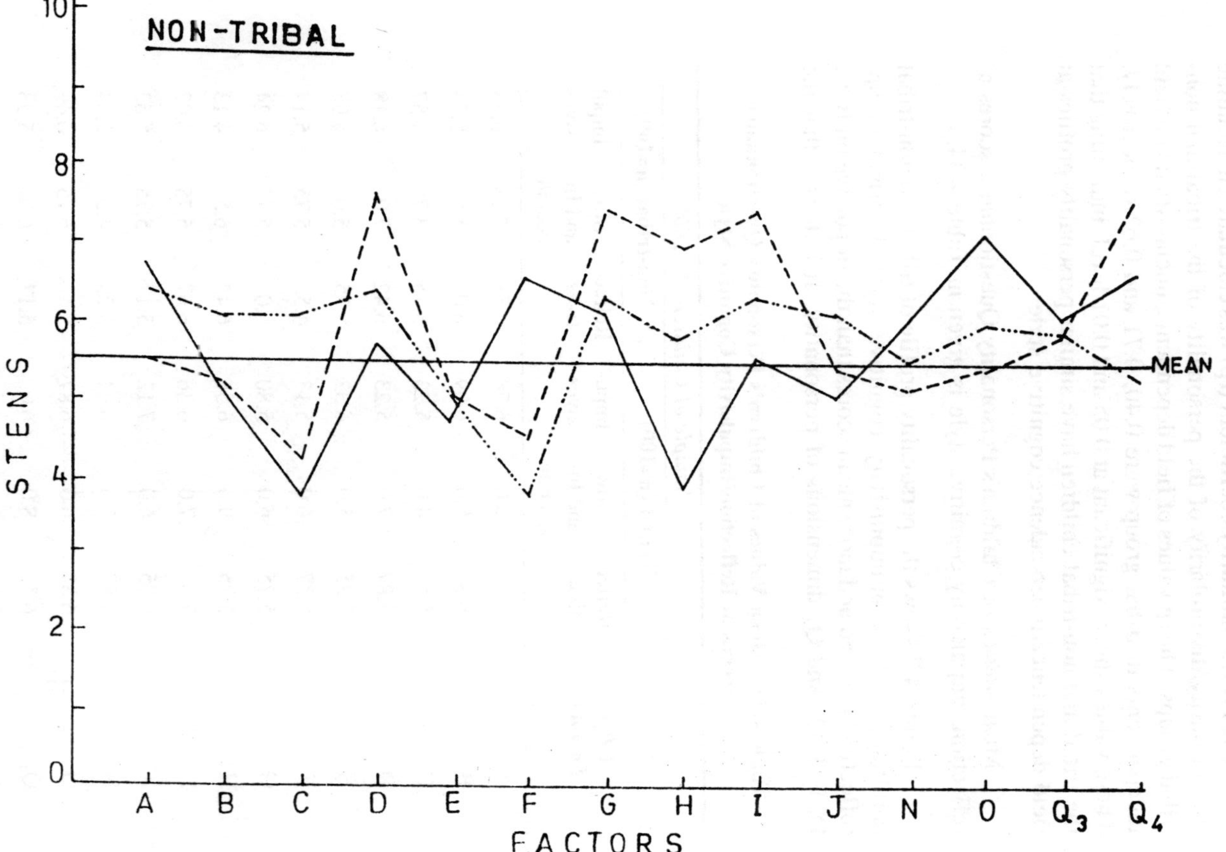

Fig. 4.6 : Personality Profile of Tribal and Non-tribal Children at Field Dependence/Independence Cognitive Style

The Profile similarity coefficient (rp) was calculated to examine the similarity/dissimilarity of the personality of the tribal and non-tribal groups, The rp values of field dependents, unclassified and field independents in tribal group were 0.40, 0.71 and 0.62 respectively. These values shows significant at 0.05 and 0.01 level, indicating that the tribal and non-tribal children have similar personality profiles at field dependence/independence cognitive style.

Mean values of Children's Personality Questionnaire scores at reflection/ impulsivity cognitive style is given in Table 4.34.

Figure 4.7 shows the personality profile of tribal and non-tribal children at reflection/impulsivity cognitive style. In tribal group, reflectively scored and more mean scores than the impulsive on B, C, D, F, I, Q_3 and Q_4 dimensions of personality. It indicates that the

Table 4.34 : Mean Values of Children's Personality Questionnaire Scores at Reflection/Impulsivity Cognitive Style

	Sample of Children (N=200)					
	Tribal (n=100)			Non-tribal (n=100)		
CPQ Factors	Reflec-tives	Slow and In-accurates	Impu-sives	Relfec-tives	Slow and In-accurates	Impul-sives
A	6.0	6.0	6.78	6.58	7.75	6.63
B	6.87	5.0	6.09	6.0	5.5	5.74
C	5.5	4.0	5.23	5.75	3.75	4.57
D	5.87	7.0	5.23	6.42	7.0	6.18
E	5.25	5.0	6.32	5.25	5.0	4.98
F	5.37	6.0	5.13	4.5	5.75	5.14
G	5.75	6.0	5.80	6.0	5.75	6.24
H	5.75	9.0	6.56	6.42	6.5	4.13
I	7.0	7.0	6.36	6.67	5.75	6.07
J	6.75	6.0	7.12	5.17	5.75	5.62
N	4.87	3.0	6.44	5.25	4.0	5.64
O	6.37	6.0	6.87	5.5	6.75	6.49
Q_3	6.5	8.0	6.0	5.17	6.0	5.93
Q_4	5.37	6.0	5.33	5.60	8.5	6.24

reflective are more intelligent, emotionally stable, excitable, happy-go-lucky, tender-minded, controlled and tense than the impulsives. Reflective also scored lower mean values on some personality factors like A, E, G, H, J, N and O than the impulsive thereby indicating that they are more reserved, humble, expedient, shy, trusting, fortnight and placid, than the impulsive. Some of the results supported by Achhpal and Mistry's (1981) study.

In non-tribal group, the reflective scored higher mean values on B, C, D, E, H and I factors than the impulsive there by pointing that they are more intelligent, emotionally stable, excitable, assertive, venturesome and tender-minded than the impulsives. Reflectives also scored lower mean scores on A, F, G, J, N, O, Q_3 and Q_4 factors than the impulsive which shows that they are more reserved, sober, expedient, trusting, fortnight, placid indisciplined, self-conflict and relaxed than impulsives.

Bannigan and Ash (1977) found that the reflective children perform significantly better on the WISC than the impulsive Similar-trend is seen i.e. reflective are more intelligent than the impulsives. Similar trend is seen in tribal and non-tribal group. The obtained Profile similarity coefficient (rp) values for reflectives, slow and inaccurates and impulsives were 0.51, 0.95 and 0.29 respectively. These rp values for reflectives and slow and inaccurates are significant at 0.01 level and for impulsives, not significant at any level. That shows tribal and non-tribal children have more similar personality profiles for reflectives and slow and inaccurates with regard to impulsives, more dissimilarity of personality profiles are seen between tribal and non-tribal children.

6. RESULTS OF MULTIPLE DISCRIMINANT FUNCTION ANALYSIS

In this section of the Multiple Discriminant Function Analysis was reported to distinguish between and tribal and non-tribal groups on the basis of a set of discriminating variables on which the groups are expected to differ.

There are various statistical techniques, like "Student t-test', Analysis of Variance and co-variance, etc. available to distinguish groups on the basis of the mean score but they fail to take into account the relative weight of information for differentiation provided by the several variables. These traditional methods also fail to take into

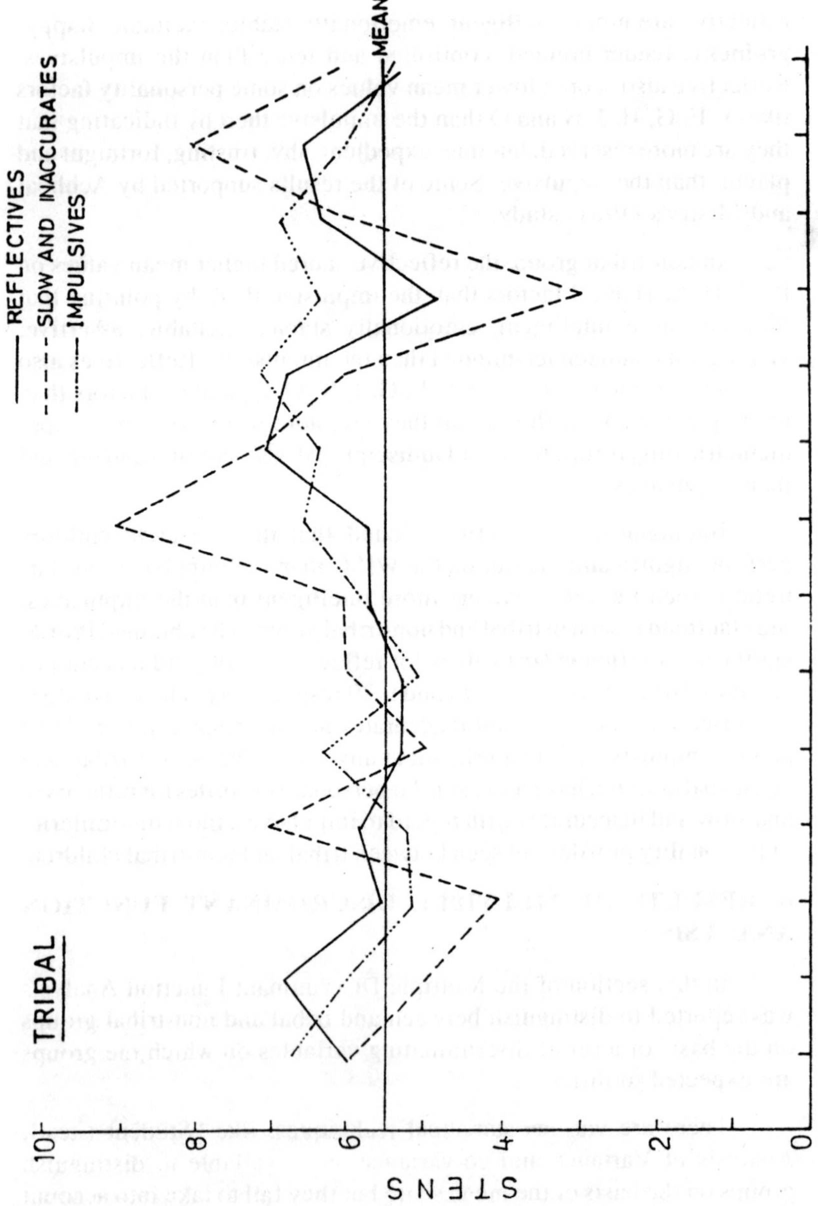

TRIBAL
REFLECTIVES
SLOW AND INACCURATES
IMPULSIVES
MEAN
10
8
6
4
2
0
STENS

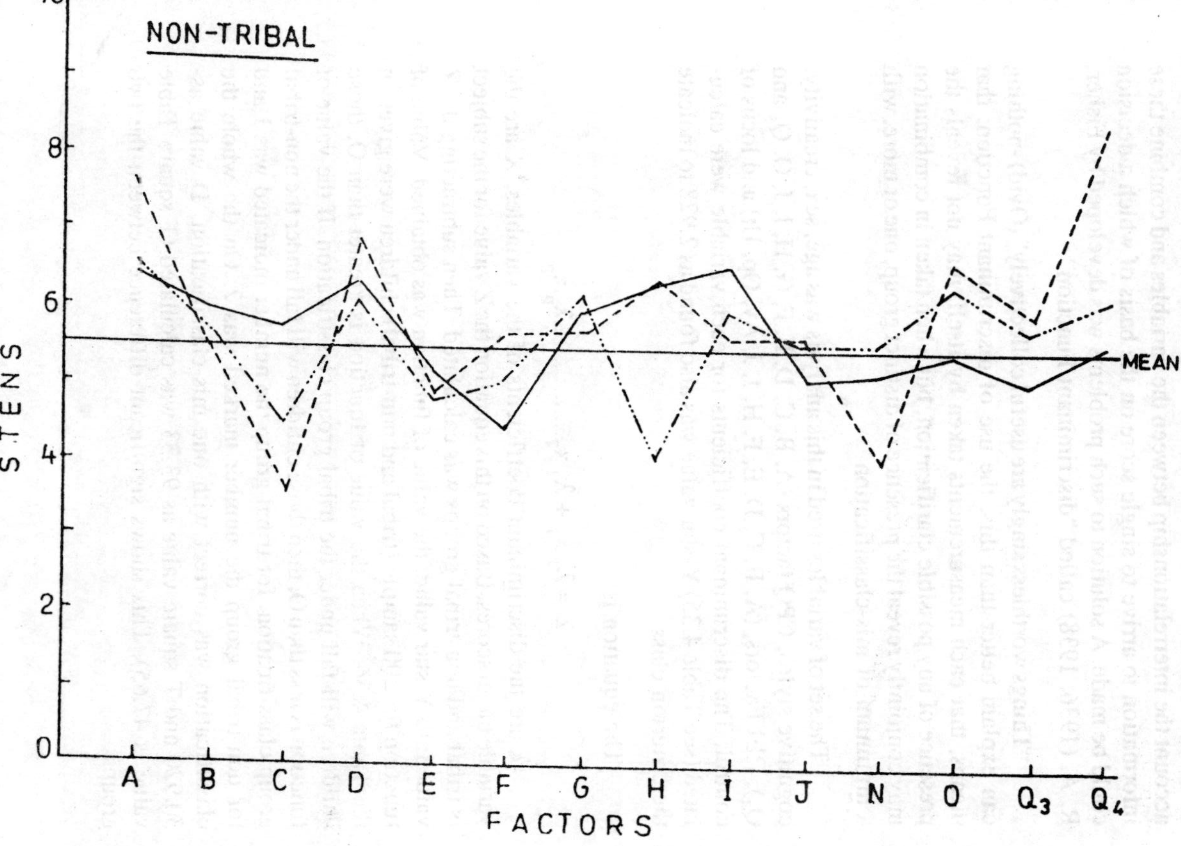

Fig. 4.7 : Personality Profile of Tribal and Non-tribal Children at Reflection/Impulsivity Cognitive Style

account the interrelationship between the variables and combine these information to arrive to single score on the basis of which a decision could be made. A solution to such problems was developed by Fisher, R. A. (1936, 1938) called "discriminant Function".

"Things worthless singly are useful collectively" (Ovid) -nothing can explain better than this, the use of discriminant Function: that means, that each measurements taken by itself, may not reveals the presence of any possible clarification, but when taken in combination may conjointly reveal the presence of distinct group, one or more, with a minimum of mis-classification.

The set of variables used in this analysis was age, sex, creativity, cognitive styles, CPQ factors (A, B, C, D, E, F, G, H, I, J, O, Q_3 and Q_4), HEI Factors, (A, B, C, D, E, F, H, I, J, Av, Op, Ut) and locus of control. The discriminant coefficients for each variable were calculated (see Table 4.35) Y-star value was also found as 2.928 to indicate the criterion class.

The equation is

$$Z = \lambda_1 x_1 + \lambda_2 x_2 \ldots\ldots\ldots\ldots\ldots \lambda_p x_p$$

λ are the discriminant coefficients of the variables, X are the variable mean scores. Based on this equation the Z value for the subject is tribal and non-tribal groups was calculated. Then subtracting the Z value into Y-star value, the value of function was obtained. Value of function for 200 sample (tribal and non-tribal) children were given in the Table 4.36. When the value of function is greater than O, those children will fall under the tribal group classification. If the value of function is less than O, then those children will fall under the non-tribal group classification. for tribal group the number indicated was 1 and for non-tribal group the number marked was 2. On the whole the classification was correct with one mis-classification. D value as-30.920 and T square value as 93.33 was calculated (T square Table value is 47.65). This shows significant difference between the two groups.

Table 4.35 : Discriminant Co-efficients of Variables Used in Multiple Discriminant Functional Analysis

S. No.	*Variable*	*Discriminant Coefficients (T)*
1.	Age	–0 .077
2.	Sex	0.264
3.	Creativity	0.494
4.	Cognitive Styles	–0.039
	CPQ Factors	
5.	A	0.319
6.	B	–0.382
7.	C	0.842
8.	D	–0.185
9.	E	–0.382
10.	F	–0.164
11.	G	0.426
12.	H	0.138
13.	I	–0.433
14.	J	–0.028
15.	N	–0.150
16.	O	–0.258
17.	Q3	0.025
18.	Q4	–0.118
	HEI Factors	
19.	A	0.257
20.	B	0.501
21.	C	0.279
22.	D	–0.039
23.	E	–0.216
24.	F	0.226
25.	G	–0.041
26.	H	0.085
27.	I	0.173
28.	J	0.371
29.	Av	–0.043
30.	Op	–0.210
31.	Ut	0.260
32.	Locus of control	–0.761

Table 4.36 : Value of Functions for Sample Children

Subjects	*Value of Function*	*Classification* *1–Tribal Group* *2-Non-tribal Group*
1.	2.300	1
2.	2.075	1
3.	1.219	1
4.	0.441	1
5.	2.159	1
6.	2.176	1
7.	0.941	1
8.	0.330	1
9.	1.843	1
10.	1.446	1
11.	1.045	1
12.	0.541	1
13.	1.105	1
14.	1.582	1
15.	1.087	1
16.	1.528	1
17.	1.236	1
18.	1.590	1
19.	1.767	1
20.	1.784	1
21.	1.858	1
22.	0.335	1
23.	0.572	
24.	0.863	1
25.	1.180	1
26.	2.107	1
27.	0.918	1
28.	0.831	1
29.	1.282	1
30.	1.765	1

Contd.

Table 4.36 : (Contd.)

Subjects	*Value of Function*	*Classification 1–Tribal Group 2-Non-tribal Group*
31.	0.628	1
32.	1.498	1
33.	1.372	1
34.	1.615	1
35.	1.846	1
36.	0.941	1
37.	0.978	1
38.	1.209	1
39.	1.205	1
40.	0.816	1
41.	1.297	1
42.	1.418	1
43.	0.412	1
44.	0.415	1
45.	0.658	1
46.	1.231	1
47.	0.867	1
48.	1.128	1
49.	0.578	1
50.	0.863	1
51.	0.652	1
52.	0.496	1
53.	0.583	1
54.	1.114	1
55.	0.927	1
56.	1.135	1
57.	0.889	1
58.	0.795	1
59.	1.563	1
60.	1.181	1

Contd.

Table 4.36 : (Contd.)

Subjects	Value of Function	Classification 1–Tribal Group 2-Non-tribal Group
61.	1.032	1
62.	1.014	1
63.	1.265	1
64.	0.897	1
65.	1.589	1
66.	0.289	1
67.	0.409	1
68.	0.266	1
69.	0.251	1
70.	0.676	1
71.	0.341	1
72.	0.361	1
73.	0.475	1
74.	0.707	1
75.	0.385	1
76.	0.327	1
77.	1.015	1
78.	0.584	1
79.	0.361	1
80.	1.154	1
81.	0.489	1
82.	0.306	1
83.	–0.647	2
84.	0.633	1
85.	0.251	1
86.	0.306	1
87.	0.688	1
88.	0.602	1
89.	0.833	1
90.	0.768	1

Contd.

Table 4.36 : (Contd.)

Subjects	*Value of Function*	*Classification 1–Tribal Group 2-Non-tribal Group*
91.	0.680	1
92.	0.751	1
93.	0.315	1
94.	0.273	1
95.	0.708	1
96.	0.636	1
97.	0.378	1
98.	1.199	1
99.	0.125	1
100.	0.389	1
101.	–0.910	2
102.	–0.680	2
103.	–1.069	2
104.	–0.531	2
105.	–1.024	2
106.	–1.708	2
107.	–0.874	2
108.	–1.109	2
109.	–1.509	2
110.	–1.296	2
111.	–0.746	2
112.	–1.192	2
113.	–1.553	2
114.	–1.227	2
115.	–0.715	2
116.	–1.017	2
117.	–0.777	2
118.	–1.192	2
119.	–1.082	2
120.	–1.506	2

Contd.

Table 4.36 : (Contd.)

Subjects	*Value of Function*	*Classification 1–Tribal Group 2-Non-tribal Group*
121.	–0.987	2
122.	–0.881	2
123.	–1.102	2
124.	–1.135	2
125.	–0.991	2
126.	–1.157	2
127.	–0.971	2
128.	–0.905	2
129.	–0.992	2
130.	–1.235	2
131.	–0.986	2
132.	–1.371	2
133.	–1.129	2
134.	–1.332	2
135.	–1.529	2
136.	–0.612	2
137.	–0.629	2
138.	–0.592	2
139.	–0.602	2
140.	–1.027	2
141.	–1.497	2
142.	–1.000	2
143.	–0.866	2
144.	–1.072	2
145.	–0.796	2
146.	–0.909	2
147.	–0.863	2
148.	–1.023	2
149.	–0.756	2
150.	–1.199	2

Contd.

Table 4.36 : (Contd.)

Subjects	*Value of Function*	*Classification 1–Tribal Group 2-Non-tribal Group*
151.	–0.975	2
152.	–1.037	2
153.	–0.577	2
154.	–0.610	2
155.	–0.857	2
156.	–0.603	2
157.	–0.424	2
158.	–0.983	2
159.	–1.102	2
160.	–0.888	2
161.	–0.793	2
162.	0.491	2
163.	–1.063	2
164.	–1.440	2
165.	–1.503	2
166.	–0.287	2
167.	–0.805	2
168.	–0.972	2
169.	–0.852	2
170.	–0.952	2
171.	–0.483	2
172.	–0.748	2
173.	–0.607	2
174.	–0.864	2
175.	–0.637	2
176.	–0.540	2
177.	–0.986	2
178.	–0.821	2
179.	–0.912	2
180.	–0.709	2

Contd.

Table 4.36 : (Contd.)

Subjects	*Value of Function*	*Classification 1–Tribal Group 2-Non-tribal Group*
181.	–0.462	2
182.	–1.032	2
183.	–1.246	2
184.	–0.680	2
185.	–0.864	2
186.	–0.469	2
187.	–0.851	2
188.	–1.009	2
189.	–1.263	2
190.	–1.217	2
191.	–1.133	2
192.	–0.809	2
193.	–0.419	2
194.	–1.077	2
195.	–1.051	2
196.	–1.029	2
197.	–0.434	2
198.	–0.966	2
199.	–1.118	2
200.	–0.660	2

	Correct Classification	Mis-Classification
Tribal subjects (1–100)	99	1
Non-Tribal Subjects (1–200)	100	0

From the data presented in preceding page, it is interesting to note that the variables taken in this analysis were discriminated well.

5

SUMMARY

The main thrust of the investigation is to study how certain demographic (ethnicity, age and sex), psychological (personality and locus of control) and environmental (home environment) factors contribute to the expression of creativity and the cognitive styles in Sugali tribal and non-tribal children.

RESEARCH QUESTIONS

For the study, the following research questions were framed:

1. **Is there is a significant relationship between creativity and cognitive styles?**
2. **In what way and how some of the important demographic (ethnicity, age and sex), psychological (personality and locus of control) and environmental (home environment) factors influence the expression of creativity and cognitive styles ?**
3. **Is there a different incidence of verbal and non-verbal components of creativity among the tribal and non-tribal children?**
4. **Out of the two cognitive styles (field dependence/independence and reflection/impulsivity), which cognitive style is predominantly seen in tribal and non-tribal children ?**

The review of literature related to the topic was presented in the following scheme.

1. Contributions to the measurement of creativity and cognitive styles.
2. Studies on inter-relation between creativity and cognitive styles.
3. Influence of demographic factors on creativity and cognitive styles.
4. Influence of psychological factors on creativity and cognitive styles.
5. Influence of psychological factors on creativity and cognitive styles.

On the whole, the review of literature with regard to creativity and cognitive styles with different variables has revealed certain inconsistent and inconclusive results that necessitate the present study.

Ethnographic profile on Sugali tribe of Chittoor district includes their origin, economy, occupation, income housing, and living condition, household possessions, racial features, languages and literacy, groups, names dress pattern, ornaments, food habits, social customs, law and justice, marriage, practices, types of family and child rearing practices was given in Methodology chapter.

RESEARCH TOOLS USED

The selected research tools are as follows:

1. Mehdi's (1973) Test of Verbal and Non-verbal Creative Thinking to measure creativity (adapted by the Investigator);
2. Embedded Figures Test to measures field independence/ independence cognitive style;
3. Matching Familiar Figures Test to measure reflection/ impulsivity cognitive style (developed by the Investigator);
4. Adapted version of Children's personality questionnaire (Siddamma, 1979) to assess children's personality (modified by the Investigator);

5. Rotter's (1966) Internal and Control Scale to measure locus of control (adapted and modified by the Investigator);
6. Adapted version of Home Environment Inventory (Manjuvani and Kalyani, 1987) to assess home environment (modified by the Investigator).

The description, development, adaptation and modification of the tools used in the study, reliability and validity of the tools and scoring procedure were clearly explained in Methodology chapter.

SAMPLE FOR FINAL STUDY

The Investigator selected a comparable group of 100 Sugali tribal and 100 non-tribal children of both sexes representing 10,11 and 12 years age group (5th, 6th and 7th standards) form Punganur, Madanapalli and Piler Mandals of Chittoor district in Andhra Pradesh.

DATA COLLECTION

The required data were collected from the studies directly through the administration of different tests prepared for the purpose. Administration was done according to the procedure and instructions given in test booklets and manuals.

The obtaining data were analysed by using appropriate statistical techniques i.e., Percentages, chi-square Analysis, t-test, F-test, Correlation coefficients, Multiple Regression Analysis, Personality Profiles and Discriminant Function Analysis.

FINDINGS AND CONCLUSIONS

Number of Children in Different Levels of Creativity:

1. High percentage (49%) on non-tribal children are identified as high creativity in verbal creativity as compared to the tribal children. In other words, the tribal children are deficient with regard to the level of verbal creative thinking.
2. The equal number of high creativity (43%) are identified in tribal and non-tribal children. It means tribal children's performance in non-tribal creative measures is similar to that of the non-tribal children.
3. The chi-square analysis reveals that there is no significant

association between high, average and low creatives and verbal and non-verbal creativity in tribal and non-tribal children.

4. **Many of tribal boys (53.33%) with 11 years age are classified as high creativity in both verbal and non-verbal creativity. Whereas, many of tribal girls in the same age group have exhibited low verbal (53.33%) and non-verbal (46.67) creativity.**

5. **In the non-tribal 11 years age group, many for the boys and girls (53.33%) are classified as low creatives in verbal and non-verbal creativity. Many of the non-tribal boys with 12 years age are identified as high creatives in verbal (57.89%) and non-verbal (47.37%) components of creativity. Half of the girls in this age showed high creatives in verbal and more than half as low creatives in non-verbal creativity.**

Number of Children Showing Different Cognitive Styles

1. Higher percentage (51%) of tribal children are field dependent and relatively higher percentage (55%) non-tribal children are field independents. With regard to reflection/ impulsivity cognitive styles, higher percentage of tribal children (91%) and non-tribal children (84%) are impulsives.

2. The chi-square analysis reveals that there is no statistically significant association between field dependents, field independents and unclassified and tribal and non-tribal groups. Also, it is noticed that there is no significant association between reflectives, impulsives and slow and inaccurates and tribal and non-tribal groups.

3. In the age group of 10 years, many of the tribal boys (83.33%) and girls (88.23%) are field dependents. The percentage of field dependents among boys and girls in the age group of 11 years is low when compared to the 10 years age group. Higher percentage of boys (94.7%) and girls (81.25%) as seen as field independents in 12 years age group.

4. Most of the non-tribal boys (88.89%) and girls (98.12%) are field dependents in 10 years age group. More than half of the boys and girls field independents in 11 years age

group. In the 12 years age group greater percentage is considered field independents.

5. Irrespective of age, a few tribal boys and girls are classified as reflectives. Most of the boys and girls are found to be impulsives in 10 years and 12 years age group when compared to 11 years age group.

6. In the 12 years age group of non-tribal, the reflectives are found more in number than in the 11 years age group. In other words, when age increases, the presence of reflection cognitive style also increases and impulsivity cognitive a style decreases.

Difference between Tribal and Non-Tribal Children on Dependent and Independent Variables.

1. Non-tribal children excel the tribal children in the verbal components of creativity. There is no significant difference between tribal and non-tribal children with regard to non-verbal creativity.

2. The difference in performance between the successive age groups is significant for all verbal and non-verbal components of creativity measures in tribal and non-tribal children.

   In tribal group, when age increased the verbal and non-verbal components of creativity also increased. Whereas in non-tribal group, 11 years of age group children showed lower level of performance than the 10 years age group in all verbal components of creativity except elaboration component. In non-verbal creativity only originality component showed lower level of performance than the 10 years age group.

   On the whole, the 12 years age group obtained the highest mean values in verbal and non-verbal components of creativity in tribal and non-tribal children.

3. Statistically, significant differences are found with respect of boys and girls in all verbal except elaboration component and non-verbal components of creativity in tribal children. In the non-tribal group significant differences are seen with regard to boys and girls in all verbal and non-verbal

components of creativity.

4. Field dependence/independence cognitive style is mostly seen in tribal children when compared to the non-tribal children. The reflection/impulsivity cognitive style is equally seen in tribal and non-tribal children.
5. When the children's age increases in tribal and non-tribal groups, the field/dependence/independence cognitive style decreases. In the case of reflection/impulsivity cognitive style, the increasing trend is observed when age increases.
6. There are less significant differences of field dependence/independence cognitive style scores in both tribal and non-tribal groups according to sex. In the case of reflection/impulsivity cognitive style, there is no significant difference with respect of sex in both tribal and non-tribal groups.
7. The mean values of A, B, F, H, I, N, O, Q_3 and Q_4 CPQ factors in tribal and non-tribal children are not significantly different. The remaining factors like C, D, E, G and J showed remarkable differences between tribal and non-tribal children.

The calculated profile similarity co-efficient value (rp) is significant at 0.01 level indicating more similarity of the personality factors among tribal and non-tribal children.

8. It is evident that CPQ factors like A, B, C, E, F, G, H, I, J and N in tribal children and D, E, G, H, N and Q_3 in non-tribal children showed statistically non significant differences according to the age levels (10, 11 and 12 years). Remaining factors like D, O, Q and Q tribal children and A, B, C, F, I, J, O and Q in non-tribal children showed significant differences by age levels.

   The obtained rp values are significant at 0.01 levels indicating more similarity between the personality factors of tribal and non-tribal children by age.

9. It is evident that the mean scores of A and E CPQ factors in tribal and A and D factors in non-tribal children differ significantly according to sex. Looking into the remaining factors, with regard to mean scores of tribal and non-tribal children, no significant differences are seen on the basis of sex

The calculated rp values are significant at 0.01 level indicating that the two groups of children have similar personality pattern by sex.

10. There is no significant difference with regard to locus of control (I-E) score between tribal and non-tribal children.
11. There is no significant difference with regard to locus of control (I-E) score between tribal and non-tribal children on the basis of age levels i.e., 10,11, and 12 years.
12. The mean value of locus of control (I–E) score in tribal boys and girls is not significantly different. On the other hand, in the non-tribal group, the locus of control (I–E) score in boys and girls showed no significant differences.
13. The mean scores of HEI factors like B,C, D, F, Av, Op and Ut between tribal and non-tribal children are significantly different. Other factors like A, E, G, H, I and J are not significantly different between tribal and non-tribal children. On the whole, the total Home Environment Inventory mean score for tribal group is higher than the non-tribal group. The results imply the existence of a good home environment in tribal group compared to the non-tribal group.
14. In the tribal group, the mean values of A, B, E, F, H, J, and Ut HEI factors and in non-tribal group, the mean values of F, H, J, Av and Op factors differed significantly with respect to their different age levels.
15. Only I factor in tribal and A, G, Op and Ut factors in non-tribal children showed significant differences on the basis of sex.

Relationship between Creativity and Cognitive Styles

1. In the tribal and non-tribal groups, the verbal and non-verbal creativity are negatively correlated with field dependence/independence cognitive style. In other words, there is significant correlation between creativity and field independence cognitive style.
2. In the tribal group, the verbal and non-verbal creativity is not significantly correlated with reflection/impulsivity cognitive style. In the non-tribal group, only verbal creativity

is significantly and positively correlated with reflection/ impulsivity cognitive style. In other words, there is significant correlation between verbal creativity and reflection cognitive style.

Multiple (Step-wise) Regression Analysis

1. When total verbal creativity scores of tribal children were treated as the dependent variable, age, sex, scores of cognitive styles (field dependence/independence and reflection/impulsivity), total HEI and locus of control (I-E) score of tribal children were considered independent variables, only age and sex were entered. These two variables put together could explain about 38.6 per cent (R=0.386) of the variance in the dependent variable, verbal creativity. Out of this 23.8 per cent of the variance was explained by age and the remaining 14.8 per cent by sex.
2. When the total non-verbal creativity scores of tribal children were treated as the dependent variable, age, sex, scores of cognitive styles (field dependence/independence and reflection/impulsivity), total HEI score and locus of control (I-E) score of tribal children were computed as independent variables; only age and sex were entered. These two variables put together could explain about 33.9 per cent (R^2=0.339) of the variance in the dependent variable, non-verbal creativity. Out o this 27.1 per cent accounted for age and the remaining 6.8 per cent was explained by sex.

Inter-correlations among Independent variables and their correlation with dependent variable:

In the tribal group, among the independent variables, only age factors shows significant negative correlation with field dependence/ independence cognitive style and locus of control.

A significant positive correlation was seen between verbal and non-verbal creativity and age variable.

A significant negative correlation was observed between verbal and non-verbal creativity and sex, field dependence/independence and locus of control.

3. When total verbal creativity scores of non-tribal children were treated as the dependent variable, age, sex, scores of cognitive styles (field dependence/independence and reflection/impulsivity), total HEI score and locus of control (I-E) score of non-tribal children as the independent variables, only age and sex were entered. The percentage variance in creativity (verbal) explained by these two variables viz., age and sex was 38.9 (R^2=0.389). Out of this 32.3 per cent and 6.6 per cent of variance were accounted for by age and sex respectively.
4. When the total non-verbal creativity scores of non-tribal children were treated as the dependent variable, age, sex, scores of cognitive styles (field dependence/independence), total HEI scores and locus of control (I-E) score of non-tribal children as the independent variables, only age and sex were entered. The value of R^2 (0.323) disclosed that the two variables put together could explain about 32.3 per cent of the variance in the dependent variable, non-verbal creativity. Out of this, 26.3 per cent was accounted for by age and the remaining 6.0 per cent was explained by sex.

Inter-correlations among Independent variables and their correlation with dependent variable.

In the non-tribal groups, there is significant negative correlation between age and field dependence/independence cognitive style. Age also significantly showed positive correlation with reflection/impulsivity cognitive style.

The sex variable has significant negative correlation with total Home Environment Inventory score.

Field dependence/independence cognitive style is significantly negatively correlated with reflection/impulsivity cognitive style.

A significant positive correlation was seen between verbal creativity and age, reflection/impulsivity cognitive style and home environment.

A negative significant correlation was found between verbal creativity and sex and field dependence/independence cognitive style.

The significant positive correlation was found with age, significant negative correlation was with sex and field dependence/independence cognitive styles.

5. When the field dependence/independence cognitive style scores of tribal children were treated as the dependent variable, age, sex, creativity (verbal and non-verbal) score, total HEI score and locus of control (I-E) score of tribal children as independent variables, only age and sex were entered. These two variables put together could explain about 56.4 per cent (R^2=0.564) of the variance in the dependent variable. Out of this, 53.7 per cent of the variance was explained by age and the remaining 2.7 per cent of the variance was explained by sex.
6. When cognitive style (reflection/impulsivity) scores of tribal children were tribal as the dependent variable, there was no independent variable entered in the Multiple Regression Analysis.

Inter-correlations among Independent variables and their correlation with dependent variables:

In the tribal groups significant positive correlation exists between age and verbal and non-verbal creativity. Age also significantly and negatively correlated with locus of control.

There is highly negative correlation between sex variable and verbal and non-verbal creativity.

Verbal creativity is positively correlated with non-verbal creativity. Verbal and non-verbal creativity is negatively correlated with locus of control.

Field dependence/independence cognitive style is highly cognitive correlated with age, verbal creativity and non-verbal creativity.

With regard to reflection/impulsivity cognitive style, no significant correlation was found with any independent variable.

7. When total field dependence/independence cognitive style scores of non-tribal children were treated as the dependent variable, age, sex, creativity score (verbal and non-verbal) total HEI score and locus of control (I-E) score of non-tribal children as independent variables, only age and sex were entered. The value of R^2 (0.681) disclosed that 68.1 per cent of variance on field dependence/independence cognitive

style was explained by two variable. The variance contributed by age and sex are 64.9 per cent and 3.2 per cent respectively.

8. When the cognitive style (reflection/impulsivity) scores of non-tribal children were treated as the dependent variable, age, sex, creativity score (verbal and non-verbal), total HEI score and locus of control (I-E) score of non-tribal children as the independent variables, only age was entered. The R^2 disclosed that about 20.8 per cent of the variance in cognitive style (reflection/impulsivity) was accounted for by age alone. The other independent variable was not entered which means that it did not influence the cognitive style (reflection/impulsivity) of the non-tribal children.

Inter-correlations among Independent variables and their correlation with dependent variable:

In the non-tribal group, the highly significant correlation was seen between age and verbal and non-verbal creativity.

Negative correlation was found between sex and verbal and non-verbal creativity. Sex is also negatively correlated with home environment.

Verbal and non-verbal creativity are significantly positively correlated and they bothare positively related to home creativity.

Field dependence/independence cognitive style has highly significant negative correlation with age, verbal and non-verbal creativity.

With reference to reflection/impulsivity cognitive style, there is highly significant positive relationship with age and verbal creativity.

Personality Profiles

1. In the tribal group, the mean scores of high creative children are more than the mean score of the low creative children on A, B, C, D, F, G, H, I, J, N, O and Q_3 dimension of personality. High creatives scored lower mean values than the low creativity on E and Q_4 dimension of personality.

In the non-tribal group, the mean scores of high creative children are more than the low creative children on A, D, F, H, I, N and O dimensions of personality.

Equal mean scores were obtained for the high and the low creatives on B, E and J factors. High creatives scored lower mean scores the low creatives on C, E, G, Q and Q factors.

The obtained rp values (significant at 0.05 level) with regard to verbal creativity indicates that the high creatives in tribal and non-tribal groups had similar personality profiles. For average creatives the rp was not significant. It shows the dissimilarity of personality profiles. With respect of the low creatives, the rp values is significant at 0.01 level indicating that low creatives in tribal and non-tribal groups have more similar personality profiles.

2. In the tribal group, the mean scores of high creatives are greater than the mean scores of low creative group on A, F, H and N dimensions of personality. High creatives scored similar mean values as low creatives on G and Q_3 factors. High creatives also scored lower mean scores on B, C, D, E, I, J, O and Q_3 than the low creatives.

In the non-tribal group, the mean scores of high creative children are more than mean scores of low creative children on A, B, C, D, E, F, G, I, N and Q_3. High creatives obtained lower mean scores than the low creatives on H, J, O and Q_4 dimensions of personality. In non-verbal creativity with regard to high creatives the profile similarity co-efficient (rp value) was significant at 0.01 level which shows that the high creatives on tribal and non-tribal groups have more similar personality profiles. For the average and low creatives, the obtained rp values were not significant. It shows the dissimilarity of personality profiles in tribal and non-tribal group.

3. In the tribal group, the field dependents scored higher mean scores on B, E, F, G, J, N and O factors than the field independents. Field dependents also scored lower mean scores on A, C, D, H, I, Q and Q than the field independents.

In non-tribal group, the field dependents scored more mean values on, A, F, N, O, Q_3 and Q_4 factors than the field independents. They also scored lower mean values on B, C, D, G, H, I and J dimensions of personality than the field independents.

The profile similarity co-efficient (rp) was calculated to examine the similarity and dissimilarity of the personality of the tribal and non-tribal groups. The rp values of field dependents, unclassified and field independents in tribal group are significant at 0.05 and 0.01 level indicating that the tribal and non-tribal children have similar personality profiles at field dependence/independence cognitive style.

4. In tribal group, reflectives scored more mean scores than the impulsives on B, C, D, F, I, Q_3 and Q_4 dimensions of personality. Reflectives also scored lower mean values on score personality factors like A, E, G, H, J, N and O than impulsives.

In non-tribal group, the reflectives scored higher mean values on B, C, D, E, H and I factors than the impulsives. Reflectives also scored lower mean scores on A, F, G, J, N O, Q_3 and Q_4 factors than the impulsives.

The obtained rp values of reflectives and slow and inaccurates are significant at 0.01 level and for impulsives not significant at any level. This shows tribal and non-tribal children more similar personality profiles for reflectives and slow and inaccurates. With regard to impulsives, more dissimilarity of personality profiles are seen between tribal and non-tribal children.

Multiple Discriminant Function Analysis

1. The results of Multiple Discriminant Function analysis are reported to distinguish between tribal and non-tribal groups on the basis of a set of discriminating variables on which the groups are expected to differ.

The set of variables used in this analysis was age, sex, creativity, cognitive styles, CPQ factors (A, B, C, D, E, F, G, H, I, J, N, O, Q_3 and Q_4), HEI factors (A, B, C, D, E, F, G, H, I, J, Au, Op, Ut) and locus of control.

From the analysis, it is interesting to note that the variables taken in this were discriminated well.

Implications of the Study

1. Educators and administrators should bring about an awareness among parents to give more importance to the creative expression and different cognitive styles.
2. Parental motivation is necessary to develop creativity and cognitive styles through guiding, directing, stimulating

and encouraging the children.

3. Welfare measures should reach the tribal and non-tribal people to improve the socio-economic status as they will indirectly improve the children's proper care and opportunities by their respective parents and regular attendance in schools.
4. Understanding and co-operation between parents and teachers are necessary for smooth continuity of growth as the child moves from home into a different environment at the school. Generally parents in India think that their responsibilities will cease when they send children to school. They feel that total responsibility will be taken care of by the teachers but they do not realize that it is also their responsibility to help them in their education. Until child feels responsible, parents should shoulder the responsibility to stimulate the children to learn good habits of reading, writing, speaking, thinking and problem-solving.
5. The schools should play an important role in fostering creativity and cognitive styles of children by making the whole system of education need based and action oriented.
6. Most of the programmes in school are heavily planned towards information content rather than creative and cognitive oriented. Therefore, there is a need to review and modify the programmes in schools.
7. Educational programmes in the tribal and rural areas need to be strengthened to lay a solid foundation for their cognitive development. The programme must be interesting and suited to the culture.
8. The role of a teacher is to motivate children to accept them and to guide the childrens' learning. The stimulation by teacher is need which directly influence the children's cognitive development.
9. It is desirable to include basic aspects of creativity and cognitive styles in the teacher training programme, because the teachers are not well equipped to deal with creative thinking and cognitive styles. Periodical workshops and seminars should be organized for teachers to make them aware of latest developments in the area of

cognitive development. The national and state level educational institutions like National Council of Educational Research and Training and State Council of Educational Research and Training should take the lead and modify the existing teacher training programmes.

Limitations

1. The study is limited only to the Sugali tribal and non-tribal children in Chittoor District, Andhra Pradesh.
2. The present study considered only the factors such as demographic (ethnicity, age and sex), psychological (personality and locus of control) and environmental (home environment) to see their influence on creativity and cognitive style.
3. The sample consist of only 100 tribal and 100 non-tribal children selected from Chittoor District, Andhra Pradesh.
4. The children with 10,11 and 12 years age group are only considered in the present study.

Suggestions for Further Research

1. Investigations covering other age groups which were not included in the present study may be fruitful, because, as assessment of creativity and cognitive style on larger scale covering children of all age groups will help educationists to locate difficult areas and strengthen education programme accordingly.
2. Intra-tribal comparisons can be carried out by including other tribal group children in different parts of India.
3. Studies involving other factors which were not studied in the present enquiry like socio-economic status, family size, ordinal position of the child, educational level of the parents, school environment, level of adjustment, mental health, academic achievement, etc. would be worthwhile as not much is known about their relation to creativity and cognitive styles.
4. The methodology used to assess the reflection/impulsivity cognitive style in this study can be taken up by other researchers to see its reliability and validity.

5. **Intervention studies can be conducted to find out the impact of enriched programme and environment.**
6. **There is need for application of such studies and also a follow up.**

REFERENCES

Achhapal, B. And Mistry, V. (1981) The cognitive style among preschoolers and it's relationship to teacher's rating on learning abilities. *Child Psychiatry Quarterly*, 14(4), 126-132.

Adejumo, D. (1979) Conceptual tempo and visual perceptual ability of some Nigerian children. *Psychological Reports*, 45, 911-916.

Adeval, G., Silverman, A.J. and McGough, W.E. (1968) MMPI findings in field dependent and field independent subjects. *Perceptual and Motor Skills*, 26, 3-8.

Agarwal, S. and Bohra, S. P. (1982) Study of the personality pattern of high and low creative children. *Child Psychiatry Quarterly*, 15(4), 136-139.

Agarwal, A. and Srivastava (1981) Significance of time perspective in reflection-impulsivity. *Psychological Studies*, 26(2), 100-103.

Agarwal,V.P. and Verma L.P. (1977) Internal-external control of high creative and low creative high school students at different levels of socio-economic status. *Journal of Creative Behaviour*, 11(2), 150.

Ahmad, M. (1969) A study of the personality correlates of creative girls at the middle schools age. M. A. disseration, Aligarh Muslim University (Unpublished).

Ahmed, S (1980) Effect of Socio- cultural disadavantage on creative thinking. *Journal of Psychological Researches*, 24 (1-2), 96–106.

Ahmed, S and Joshi, R. K. (1978) Creativity growth among disadvantages children. *Psychologia: an international Journal of Psychology in Orient*, 21(3), 161-166.

Adlous, J. (1975) The search for alternatives: Parental behaviours and children's original problem solutions. *Journal of Marriage and Family*, 37(4), 711-722. In Psychological abstracts, 56 (4), 715 (5985).

Anderson, H.H. and Anderson, G.L. (1965). A cross-rational study of children: a study in creativity and mental health in Gordon, I.J. (Ed.) *Human Development: Readings in Reaserch.* Glenview, 111, Scott. Foresman.

Andre, B(1965) *Caste, Class and Power*. Los Angeles: University of California Press.

Andrews, E.G. (1930) *The Development of Imagination in the Preschool Child*, University of Lowa. Studies of Character, 3, 1-6.

Ann Floyd (1976) *Cognitive Styles*. The Open University Education Studies: A second level course, Personality and Learning, Block 5. The Open University Press, Walton, Hall Malton Keynes. MK7 6AA, 9-10, 33-51.

Arastech, A.R. and Arastech, J.D. (1976) *Creativity in Human Development*. Jogn Wiley and Sons, New York.

Arora, R.K. (1985) Personality constituents and their relation: A study of intercorrelation. *Indian Jounral of Applied Psychology*, 22(1-2), 46-52.

Asha, C.B. (1978) An empirical study of the adjustment patterns of creative children in secondary schools. Ph.D. Thesis (Psychology), Kerala University.

Asha C.B. (1983) Creativity of children of working mothers. *Psychological Studies*, 28(2), 104-106.

Asifa, A. (1986) Creativity and family background of adivasi female students. *Experiments in Education*, 14,144-146.

Asifa, A. (1987) Sex and community as the determinants of creativity.

Experiments in Education, 15,218-222.

Ault, R.L. (1973) Problem solving strategies of reflective, impulsive, fast-accurate and slow-inaccurate children. *Child Development*, 44,259-266.

Ault, R., Crawford, D. and Jaffrey, W. (1975) Visual Scanning strategies of reflective, impulsive fast-accurate and slow-inaccurate children on the Mathcing Familiar Figures Test. *Child Development*, 43. 1412.-1417.

Babu, N. A. (1977) Comparative study of the personality factors of high intelligence-high creative thinkers and high intelligence low creative thinkers in secondary schools. Ph. D. Thesis, Kerala University (Unpublished).

Badarinath, S. Satyanarayana, S.B. (1979) Correlates of creative thinking of high school students. *Creativity News Letter*, 7 and 8.

Bailey, F.G. (1961) "*Tribe*" and "Caste" *in India, contributions to Indian Sociology*. The Hague: Paris Monton and Co., V,8.

Bal, S. (1988) Creativity, Cognitive style and academic achievement amongst university students. *Psychological Studies*, 33(1).

Baldwin, A.L. (1949). The effect of home environment on nursery school behaviour. *Child Development*, 20, 49-62.

Baldwin, A.L., Kalhorn, J. and Breese, F.H. (1945) Patterns of parent behaviour. *Psychological Monograph*, 1958, 3(1), 73.

Bali, S.S. (1981) Study of common personality factors of highly creative persons in different fields. Ph. D. (Education) Thesis, Kurukshetra University.

Bannigan, G.G. and Ash, T. (1977) Cognitive Tempo and WISC-performance. *Journal of Clinical Psychology*, 33:212.

Barbe (1964) Cited by Frierson, E.C. Developing creativity. *Review of Educational Research*. American Educational Research Association, 1969, XXXIX (1), 30-31.

Barclay, A, and Cusumano, D. (1967) Father absence, cross-sex identification and field dependent behaviour in male adolescents. *Child Development*, 38, 243-250.

Barron, F.(1963) *Creativity and Psychological Health*, New York. D. Van Nostrand.

Barron, F. (1969) *Creative Person and Creative Process*. Holt, Rinehart and Winston, New York.

Beach, F.A. and Jayes, J. (1954) Effects of early experience upon the behaviour of animals. *Psychological Bulletin*, 51, 239-263.

Bennett, D.H.(1956) Perception of the upright in relation to body image. The Journal of mental Science, 102, 487-506.

Bergum B.O. (1977) Undergraduate self-perceptions of creativity and independence. *Perceptual and Motor and Skills*, 144, 187-190.

Berry. J.W. (1966) Temme and Eskimo perceptual skills, *International Journal of Psychology*, 1, 207-209.

Berzonsky, M. (1974) Reflectivity, internality, and animistic thinking. *Child Development*, 45, 785-789.

Bhan, R. (1970) Social factor in creative potentiality, *Manas*, 17(2), 21-27.

Bhaskara, S. (1986) Adaptation of Passi tests of creativity to sixth standard children of Bangalore. *Experiments in Educations*, 14, 176-180.

Bhatnagar, P. and Rastogi, M.R. (1985). Cognitive style and basic ideal disparity. *Psychological Research Journal*, 9(2), 40-45.

Bhattacharya, P.S. (1961) An experimental study of artist personality. *Proceedings : 48th Indian Science Congress*, Part III (Abstract).

Bhattacharya, S.B. (1978) Interaction of Personality and creativity. Ph. D (Education) thesis, Banaras Hindu Unversity.

Bieri, J., Bradburn, W.M. and Galinsky, M.D. (1958) Sex differences in perceptual behaviour. *Journal of Personality*, 26, 1-12.

Bieri, J. and Messerley, S. (1957) Differences in perceptual and cognitive behaviour as a function of experimence type. *Journal of Consulting Psychology*, 21, 217-221.

Bill, M. (1987) An examination of development trends in field dependence among age groups of 10-21 years of age. *Perceptual and Motor Skills*. 64, 117-118.

Block, J., Block. J.H. and Harrington, D.M. (1974) Some Misgivings about the Matching Familiar Figures Test as a measure of reflection impulsivity. *Development Psychology*, 10, 611-632.

Bloomberg, M. (1967) An inquiry into the relationship betrween field independence/dependence and creativity. *Journal of Psychology*, 67, 127-140.

Bolen, L.M. and Torrance, E.P. (1978) The influence on creative thinkinig of locus of control, cooperation, and sex. *Journal of Clinical Psychology*, 34, 903-907.

Bowd, A.D. (1975) The relationship between perceptual egocentrism and field dependence in early childhood. *Journal of Genetic Psychology*, 127, 63-69.

Boykin, A.W. (1979) Psychological behavioral verve: Some theoretical explorations and empirical manisfestations. In A.W. Boykin, A.J. Franklin & J.F. Yates (Eds), *Research directions of black psychologists*, New York : Russel Sage, 351-367.

Brecher, M. and Denmark, F.L. (1969) Inernal-external locus of control and verbal fluency. *Psychological Reports*, 25, 707-710.

Brodley, F.K. (1976) The effect of frustration on the figural creative thinking of 5th grade students. *Journal of Experimental Education*, 44(3), 20-23.

Brodzinkski, D.M. (1975) The role of conceptual tempo and stimulus characteristics in children's humour development. *Developmental Psychology*, 11, 843-850.

Bronfenbrenner, U. (1989) The ecology of cognitive development; research models and fugitive findings. Paper prepared for presentation as the Keynote address for the nineteenth annual symposium of the Jean Piaget Society, Philadelphia.

Bruner, J.S. (1962) *Studies in Cognitive Growth*, New York, John Wiley.

Bruner, J.S. (1962) The conditions of creativity. In Grubes, H., Terrell, G. and Wertheimer, M. (Eds.) *Contemporary Approaches to Creative Thinking*. New Jersey, E . Cliffs: Prentice Hall.

Burgess, W.V. (1971) The analysis of teacher creativity, pupil age and pupil sex as sources of variation among elementary pupil's performance on pre and post tests on creative thinking. *Dissertation Abstracts International*, 32, 747.

Buriel, R. (1984) Integration with traditional Mexican-American culture and socio-cultural adjustment. In Chicano psychology (2nd ed.) New York, Academic Press, 95-130.

Burns, M.J. (1969) Selected Characteristics of Children's Individual tests of creativity. *Dissertatioin Abstracts International*, 30, 1859-A.

Burt, C. (1962) Introduction: the gifted child, in F.Z.F. Bereday and J.A. Lawerys (edn.). *The Gifted Child: The year Book of Education*, 1962, Harcourt, Brace and World, New York.

Cacha, F.B. (1971) A study of creative thinking abilities of personality factors and peer nominations of fifth grade children. *Disseration abstracts International*, 32, 1329-A.

Cairns, E. and Harbison, J.I. (1975) Impulsivity: Self-report and performance measure. *British Journal of Educational Psychology*, 45, 327-329.

Cambell, S. B. and Douglas, V.I. (1972) Cognitive Styles and responses to the threat of frustration. *Canadian Journal of Behavioural Science*, 4, 30-42.

Caring, L. (1970) The relation of cognitive style, sex and intelligence to moral judgement in children. Doctrol disseration, New York University.

Carter. J. (1983). Vision or Light: Health concerns for Afro-American Children. In G.J. Powell (Ed), *The Psychological Development of Minority Children*, New York, Bruner/Mazel, 13-25.

Cashdon, S. and Welsh, G.S. (1966) Personality correlates of creative potential in talented high school students. *Journal of Personality*, 34, 445-455.

Cattell, R.B. Eber, H.W. and Tatsuoka, M.M. (1970) *Hand Book for the Sixteen Personality Factor Questionnaire* (16PF). Institute of persoality and ability testing. Champagn Illinos.

Chadha, N.K. (1981) Creativity as a functional of intelligence, SES and sex among 12th grade schools students. *Journal of Edcuation and Psychology*, 39, 27-30.

Chandha, N.K. and Chose, P. (1985) Sex differnces in creativity risk taking, intelligence and frustration, An inferential study. *Journal of Education Research and Extension*, 21(4).

Chandha, S.K. and Sen, A.K. (1981) An investigation of the relationship between creativity, personality and vocational interest of twelth grade students of Delhi School. *Our Education*, 2, 31-37.

Chauhan, N.S. (1977) Second Stratum personality factors, sex and age (adolescence) as corelates of originality. *Indian Psychological Review*, 14(1), 16-21.

Chauhan, N.S. and Tiwari, G (1974) *Manual of Creativity Test*, Agra Psychological Research cell, Agra.

Coates, S.W. (1972) *Pre-school embedded Figures Test*, Pals Alto, CA: Consulting Psychologists Press.

Coates, S. (1974) Sex differences in field dependence/independence between the ages of 3 and 6. *Perceptual and Motor Skills*, 39, 1307-1310.

Coates, S. (1974) Sex differences in field independence among pre school children. In R.C.Friedman, R.M. Richart and R.L. Vande Wiele (Eds). *Sex Differences in Behaviour*, New York: Wiley.

Crandall, V., Katkovsky, W. and Preston, A. (1960) A cenceptual formulation for some research on children's achievement development. *Child Development*, 31, 787-799.

Crandall, V., Preston, A. and Rabson, A. (1960) Maternal reactions and the development of independence and achievement behaviour in young children. *Child Development*, 31, 243-251.

Crandall, V.C. and Lacey, B.W. (1972) Children's perceptions of Internal-External control in intellectual-academic situations and their Embedded Figures Test performance. *Child Development*, 43(40,1123.

Crandall, V.J. and Sinkeldam, C. (1964) Children's dependent and achievement behaviours in social situations and their perceptual field dependence. *Journal of Personality*, 32, 1-22.

Crutchfield, R.S. Woodworth, D.G. and Albrecht, R.E. (1958) *Perceptual Performance and the Effective Person*. Lackland Air Force Base, Texas, Personnel laboratory, Wright Air Development

Center-Tn 58-60, ASTIA Document No. Ad. 151039.

Dash, R, and Dash, A.S. (1980) A study of perceptual-motor and intellectual abilities of tribal and non-tribal pre-school children. *Proceedings of the 5th International Conference of the International Association for Cross-cultural Studies*, Bhubaneswar.

Davis, M.F. (1982) Field dependence/independence and the differentiation of self and others. *Journal of Psychology*, 11(2), 109-112.

Davis, J.K. and Frank, B.M. (1979) Learning and memory of field independent/dependent individuals. *Journal of Research in Personality*, 13, 469-471.

Davis, W.L. and Phares, E.J. (1967) Internal-external control as a determinant of information-seeking in a social influence situation, Journal of Personality, 35, 547-561.

Dawson, J.L.M. (1967) Culture and Physiological influences upon spatial-perceptual processes in West Africa. *International Journal of Phychology*, 2, 115-128.

Delgado-Gaitan, C. (1987) Tradition and transitions in the learning process of Mexican children. An ethnographic view. In G. Spindler and L. Spindler (Eds.), *Interpretive ethnography of education: At home and abroad*, Hillsdale, NJ, Erlbaum 333-359.

Dershowitz, E(1971) Jewish subcultrual patterns and psychological differentiation. *International Journal of Psychology*, C, 223-232 26, 615-621.

Devos, G.A. (Ed) (1973) *Socialization for Achievement*, Barkeley, University of California Press.

Dewing, K.(1973) Some Characteristics of the parents of creative twelve-year-olds. *Journal of Personality*, 41, 71-85.

Dharmangadan, B, (1981) Creativity in relation to sex age and local, *Psychological Studies*, 26(1), 28-33.

Diaz, (1983) Thought and two languages: The impact of bilingualism on cognitive development. In E. Gordon (Ed). *Review of Research in Education*, Vol. 10, Washington, DC: American Educational Research Association.

Douing, 'K' (1970) Some correlates of creativity performance in seventh grade children. *Australian Journal of Psychology* 22(3), 269-276.

Doyle, M. (1970) A comparative study of creativity in Negroes and Concasians. *Child Study Journal*, Vol. 1(1), 25-27.

Drevdahl, J.E. (1964) Some development and environmental factors in creativity. In Taylor, C.W. (Ed) *Widening Horisons in Creativity*, New York: Wiley.

Drew G.C. Colquhoun, W.P. and Long. H. (1958) Effet of small doses of alcohol on a skill resembling drying. *British Medical Journal*, 2, 993-999.

Drouin D., Talbot, S. and Goulet, C. (1986) Cognitive styles of French Canadian atheletes, *Perceptual and Motor Skills*, 63(3), 1139–1142.

Dryer, A.S. and Wells, M.B. (1966) Parental values, parental control and creativity in young children. *Journal of Marriage and the Family*, 28,83-88.

Ducette, J. and Wolk, S. (1972) Locus of control and extremen behaviour, *Journal of consulting and clinical psychology*, 39, 253-258.

Duffy, R.A. (1978) An analysis of aesthetic sensitivity, creativity, artistic, potential, cognitive, personality and demographical variables on grades, 4, 6, 8, and 10. *Dissertation Abstracts International* 1, 38 (II-A) 6476.

Dyk, R.B. and Witkin, H.A. (1965) Family experiences related to the development of differentiation in children. *Child Development* 36, 31-36.

Eagle, M., Gold Berger, L, and Brietman, M. (1969) Field dependence and memory for social vs neutral and relevant vs irrelevant stimuli. *Perceptual and Motor Skills*, 29, 903-910.

Eisenman, R. and Foxman, D.J. (1970) Creativity: reported family patterns and scoring methodology, *Psychological Reports*, 26, 615-621.

Fancher, P.E.M. (1969) Problem solving strategies of children as a function of conceptual tempo. Unpublished doctoral dissertation, Vanderbilt University.

Feldman, D. (1973) Creativity, intelligence, and educatioin. *Mimeographed Report*. Yale Unversity Centre for the study of Education.

Finch, A.J. Jr and Kendall, P.C. (1979) Impulsive behaviour: From research to treatment in A.J. Finch, Jr. and Philip Kendall (Eds) *Clinical Treatment and Research in Child Psychopathology* Jamaica, N.Y. : Spectrum Publicatioins.

Finch, A. J., Pezzuti, K.A., Montogomery, L.E. and Kemp, S.R. (1974) reflection-impulsivity and academic attainment in emotionally disturbed children. *Journal of Abnormal Child Psychology*, 2, 71-74.

Fitzgibbons, D.J. and Goldberger, L. (1971) Task and social orientation: A study of field dependence "arousal" and memory for incidental material. *Perceptual and Motor Skills*, 32, 162-174.

Flavell, J. (1963) *The Development Psychology of Jean Piaget*, Princeton, N.J., Van Nostrand.

Flecther, K.R. (1968) congruence of self and ideal self in original and non-original high school seniors. *Dissertation Abstracts*, 28, 4907-A.

Flexer, B.K. and Roberge, J.J. (1983) a longitudinal investigation of field dependence/independence and the development of formal operational thought. *British Journal of Education Psychology*, 53, Part (2), 195-202.

Franks, C.M. (1956) Differences detemines parle personalite dans la percepfion visuelle de la verticalie. *Revue de psychologie appliquée*, 6, 2235-246.

Frank, B.M. and Noble, J.P. (1985) Field-indepedence/dependence and cognitive restructuring. *Journal of Personality and Social Psychology*, 47(50, 1129-1135.

Fu V.R., Moran, J.D., Swayers, J.K. and Milgram, R.M. (1983) Parental influence on creativity in pre school children. *Journal of Genetic Psychology*, 143(2), 289-291.

Fuqua, R.W., Bartsch, C.W. and Phye, G.D. (1975) An investigation of the relationship between cognitive temo and creativity in preschool age children. *Child Development*, 46, 779-782.

Gakhar, S. (1974) Creativity in relation to age and sex. *Journal of Educational Psychology*, 32, 133-139.

Gakhar, S.(1975) Intellectual and personality correlates of creativity, Ph. D. Thesis, Punjab University (Unpublished.).

Gakhar, S. (1975) and Gupta, A.K. (1977) A study of the relationship of creativity with self-concept among the school going children of 12+ in Jammu City, Ph. D. thesis, Punjab University (Unpublished).

Gakhar, S, and Joshi, J.N. (1980) Creativity within the framework of personological context. *Psychological Studies*, 25(1) 48-57.

Gardner, R.W., and Moriarty, A. (1968) *Personality Development at Pre adolescence*. Seattle University of Washington Press.

Garrett, H.E. (1966) *Statistics in Psychology and Education*. Bombay: Vakils Feffer and Simons Pvt. Ltd., 191, 223-225.

Gavurin, E.I. and Murgatroyd, D. (1973) Anagram solving and locus of control, *Psychological Reports*, 33, 402.

Gayathri and Jayapoorni, N. (1989) Enriching creative activities among primary school children. A Thesis submitted for M.Sc. Degree, Avanashilingam Deemed University, Coimbatore.

Getzels, J.M. and Jackson, P.W. (1961) Family environment and cognitive style: A study of the sources of highly intelligent and of highly creative adolescents. *American Sociological Review*, 26, 351-359.

Getzels, J.W. and Jackson, P.W. (1962) *Creativity and Intelligence: Explorations with Gifted Students*. John Wiley and Sons, New York, 293.

Ghuman, P.A. (1980) A comparative study of cognitive styles in three ethnic groups, *International Review of Applied Psychology*, 29, 75-87.

Ghurye, G.S. (1957) cited by Hutton, *Caste and Class in India*. Bombay: Popular Book Depot., P. 12, op. cit. p. 12.

Golderber and Bendich (1972) Field independence -dependence and cognitive restructuring, *Journal of Personality and Social Psychology*, 1985, 47(5), 1129-1135.

Golodenson, R.M. and Longman, P. (1984) *Dictionary of Psychology and Psychiatry*, New York and London.

Goldstein, H, and Peck, R. (1973) Maternal differentiation, father absence, and cognitive differentiation in children. *Archieves of General Psychiatry*, 29, 370-373.

Golwalkar, S. (1986) a study of scientific attitude, creativity and achievement of tribal students of Rajasthan, *Indian Dissertation Abstracts*, 17(2), 153-156.

Goodenough, D.R. (1976). The role of individual differences in field dependence as a factor in learning and memory. *Psychological Bulletin*, 83(4), 675-694.

Goodenough, D.R. and Karp, S.A. (1961) Field dependence and intellecttual functioning. *Journal of Abnormal and Social Psychology*, 63(2), 241-246.

Goodenough, D.R. Oltman, P.K. and Cox, P.W. (1987) The nature of individual differences in field dependence. *Journal of Research in Personality*, 21(1), 81-89.

Gopal A.K. (1975) certain differentiating personality variables of creative and non-creative Science and Engineering students, Ph. D. (Education) Thesis, Kurukshetra University (Unpublished).

Gordon, (1964) Cited by Dashabsky, A. (1976) *Ethnic Identity in Society*, R and Mcwally college publishing company, p.3.

Gottshaldt, K. (1970) The influence of past experience on the perception of figures. In M.D. Vernon (Ed.) *Experiments in Visual Perception* (29-44) Harmonds worth, Middles ex, England; Penguin Books (Original Work Published, 1926).

Gowan, J.C. (1967) Waht makes a gifted child creative ? Four theories. In Gowan, J.C. et al (Ed.) *Creativity: Its Educational Implication*. New York: John Wiley and Sons, 9-15.

Goyal, R.P. (1969) A study of some personality traits of creative children of middle school stage, Unpublished thesis, M.A.(Psychology),-Aligarh Muslim University.

Goyal R.P. (1973) Creativity and school climate: An Exploratory study, *Journal of Psychological Research*, 17(2), 77-80.

Goyal R.P. (1984) Personality correlates of creativity in secondary school teachers under training. *Psychological Studies*, 29(1), 1-3.

Grebow, H. (1973) The relationship of some parental variables to achievement and values in college women, *Journal of Educational Research*, 66(5), 203-209.

Griffiths, R. (1945) *A Study of Imagination in Early Childhod*. London: Kogan Paul Trench, Traubner and Co., London.

Guliford, J.P. (1956) The structure of intellect. *Psychological Bulletin*, 53, 267-293.

Guliford, J.P. (1962) Factors that aid and hinder creativity. *Teachers College Record*, 63, 380-392.

Guliford, J.P. and merrifield, P.R. (1960) *The Structure of Intellect Model: Its uses and Implications*. (Rep. Psychol, Lab, No. 24) University of Southern California : Los Angeles.

Gump, P.V. (1955) Relation of efficient of recognition of personality variables. Unpublished doctoral dissertation, University of Colorado.

Gutierrez, J., Sameoff, A.J. and Karerer, B.M. (1988) Accluration and SES effects on Mexican-American parents' concepts of Development. *Child Development*, 59, 250-255.

Hakuta, K. (1987) Degree of bilingualism and cognitive ability in mainland Puerto Rican Children. *Child Development*, 58, 1372–1388.

Hakuta, K. and Garcia, E.E. (1980). Bilingualism and education. *American Psychologist*, 44, 379\4-379.

Halpin, G., Halpin, G. and Torrance, E.P. (1973). Effect of sex, race and age on creative thinking ability of blind children. *Perceptual and Motors Skills*, 37(2), 389-390.

Hare, B.R. (1985). Re-examining the ahievement central tendency: sex differences within race and race differences within sex. In H.P. McAdoo and J.L. McAdoo (Eds), *Black Children*, Beverly Hils, CA: Sage, 139-151.

Hare, B.R. and Castenell, L.A. (1985) No place to run, no place to hide. Comparative status and future prospects of black boys. In M.B.

Spencer, G. Brookins and W. Allen (Eds.), *Beginnings: The Social and Affective Development of Black Children*, Hillsdale, NJ: Erlbaum, 201-214.

Harlow, S.D. (1967) The development of originality indicator of creative ability. *Dissertation Abstracts*, 28(6), 2094-A.

Harrison, A.O. Serafica, F. and McAddo, H. (1984) Ethnic families of color. In R.D. Parke(Ed). *The Family : Review of Child Development Research*, Chicago University of Chicago Press, 7, 329-371.

Harritte, A.J. (1987) An investigation of the relationships between cognitive style, visualization, and problem solving in eight grade males and females. Ph. D. abstract, Purdue University, P.No. 146. *Dissertation Abstracts International*, 49(8), 1989.

Hartmann, H. and Kris, E. (1945) The genetic approach in psychoanalysis, *Psychoannal Stud. Child*, 1, 11-30.

Haskins, R. and Mckinney, J.D. (1976) Relative effects of response tempo and accuracy on problem solving and academic achievement. *Child Development*, 47, 690-696.

Hassan, Q. and Akbar, A. (1973) a self and ideal self-discriptions of "high" and "low" creative undergrduate students. *Creativity News Letter*, 4, 42-44.

Heilbrin,A.B. (1971) Maternal child rearing and creativity in sons. *Journal of Genetic Psychology*, 119,175-179.

Helode, R.D. (1986) *Expressed Characteristics of Creative Persons*, 16(2), 107-117.

Holland, J.L. (1961) Creative and academic performance among telented adolescents. *Journal of Educatioinal Psychology*, 52, 136-147.

Holliday, B.G. (1985) Developmental imperative of social ecologies: Lessons Learned from black children. In H.P. McAdoo and J.L. McAdoo (Eds), *Black Children*, Beverly Hills, Ca, Sage, 53-71.

Hurlock, E.B. (1981) *Child Development*, McGraw HIll Inc., Tokyo, Japan, 592.

Huss, E.T. and Kayson, W.A. (1985) Effects of age, sex and speed of founding embedded figures. *Perceptual and Motor Skills* 61,591-594.

Hussain, M.G. (1974) Creativity and sex differences, *Psychological Studies*, 19(2), 126-129.

Hutton, J.H. (1963) *Caste in India*. Bombay, Oxford University Press, 9,50.

Irvine, S.H. and Berry, J.W. (Eds) (1986) *Human Abilities in Cultural Context*. Cambridge: Cambridge, University Press.

Iicoe, I. and Pierce-Jones, J.(1965) Divergent thinking, age and intelligence in white and negro children, *Child Development*, 35, 785-797.

Iwata, O.W. (1986) Some relationship of creativity with intelligence and pesonality variables. *Psychologia; An International Journal of Psychology in the Orient*, 11 (3-4), 211-220.

Jackson, R.L. (1968) An Investigation of the creative growth cruves of university students. *Dissertation Abstracts*, 28, 3508-A.

Jairal, G.S. and Sharma, A.K., (1980) Creativity and it's components as effected by intelligence, personality and their interaction. *Asian Journal of Psychology and Education*, 6(2), 26-32.

James, G.R. (1965) The relationship of teacher characteristics and pupil creativity. *Dissertation Abstracts International*, 25, 454-A.

Jarial, G.S. (1982) Are first born children more creative? *Psychological Reports*, 151, 316-355.

Jawa, S. (1976) A study on creativity and some of its personality and environmental correlates. Ph. D. Thesis, Delhi University (Unpublished).

Jhag, D.S. (1979) A study of personality correlates of creative children, 15+ studying science subjects, Ph.D (Education) Thesis, Bhopal University.

Johnson, R.C. and Medinnus, G.H. (1969) *Child Psychology: Behaviour and Development*. New York, John Wiley and Sons.

Joshi, R.J. (1974) a study of creativity and some personality traits of the intellectual gifted high school students, Ph. D. Thesis, M.S.

University, Baroda (Unpublished).

Kagan, J. (1965) Reflection-impulsivity and reading ability in primary grade children. *Child Development*, 36, 609-628.

Kagan, J. (1965) Impulsive and reflective children: Significance of conceptual tempo. In J.D. Krumboltz (Ed.) *Learning and the Educational Process*, Chicago: Rand and Mcnally, 133-161.

Kagan, J. (1966) Development studies in reflection and analysis. In A.H. Kidd and J.H. Revoire (Eds.) *Perceptual and conceptual Development in Children*, New York, International Universities Press.

Kagan, J. and Kogan, N (1970) Individual variation in cognitive processes. In P.H. Mussen (Ed) Carmichael's *Mannual of Child Psychology*, Vol 1, New York, Wiley.

Kagan, S. Lawrence, G.Z. (1982) Generalized material reinforcement and children's reading achievement, math achievement, and field independence. *The Journal of Genetic Psychology*, 141, 93-104.

Kagan, J., Pearson, L and Welch, L. (1966) Conceptual impulsivity and inductive reasoning. *Child Development*, 37, 583-594.

Kaltsounis, B, (1971) Differences in creative thinking of black anc white deaf children, *Perceptual and Motor Skills*, 32(1), 243-248.

Karp, S.A. and Konstadt, N.L. (1971) Children's Embedded Figures Test. In H.A. Witkin, P.K. Oltman, E, Raskin and S.A. Karp (Eds), *A Manual for the Embedded Figures Tests*, Palo Alto, CA: Constulting Psychologists Press, 21-26.

Kato, N.A. (1965) Fundamental study of Rod-Frame-Test, *Japanese Psychological Research*, 7, 21-26.

Kato, N.A. (1975) The relationship between cognitive style and creativity in seventh grade children. *Dissertation Abstracts International*, 36, 1509.

Kelley, G.R. (1965) Creativity, school attitude and intelligence relationships ingrades four six and eight, *Dissertation Abstracts*, 25, 6300.

Kershner, J.R. and Ledger, G. (1985) Effect of Sex intelligence, and style of thinking on creativity: A comparison of gifted and IQ children. *Journal of Personality and Social Psychology*, 48(2), 1033-1039.

Ketkar, S.V.(1903) cited by Hutton, *History of Caste in India*. New York: Itkota p. 15, Op. Cit., p 20.

Khire, U.S. (1971) Creativity in relation to intelligence and personality factors, Ph. D. Thesis, Poona University (Unpublished).

Kishore, G. (1981) A developmental study of creativity in relation to certain personality corrlates, Ph. D. (Psychology) Thesis, Aligarh Muslim University.

Klein, G.A. Blockovich, R.N., Buchalter, P.S. and Huyghe, L. (1976) Relationship between reflection-impulsivity and problem-solving. *Perceptual and Motor skills*, 42,67-73.

Kloss, M.G. (1972) The relation between adolescent creativity and selected variables, sex, adjustment, art-science preference, complexity-simplicity and type of school, *Dissertation Abstracts International*. 33, 2324-B.

Koestler, A, (1964) The act of creation. NYC: Dell cited by Olmo, B.G. in Retroduction: The key to creativity, *Journal of Creative Behaviour*, 1977, 11(3), 216-221.

Kogan, N(1973) Creativity and cognitive style: A life span perspective. In P. B. Baltes and K.W. Schaie(Eds), *Life-span Development Psychology, Personality and Socialization,* New York, Academic Press.

Kogan, N.(1977) Sex differences in creativity and cognitive styles. In S. Messick(Ed.), *Individuality in Learning: Cognitive Styles and creativity for Human Development*. San Francisco: Joseybass.

Komarik, E.(1972) *Creativity and Orthogonal factors of Personality* (Slok) Sbornik Praci-filosofici fakulty Brenske University 20 (17), 115-124.

Kopfstein, D. (1973) Risk Taking behaviour and cognitive style. *Child Development*, 44,190-192.

Koske, G.L. (1977) The adivasi child. *Home Science,* XV, 9, 6-7.

Kris, E. (1952) *Psychoanalytic Explorations in Art*, New York :

International Universities Press.

Krishna Kumari, P., Lalitha and Paramaji, S.(1986). Creative abilites of tribal children. *Educational India*, 52(BO), 103-105.

Kumar, D. (1975) An experimental study of problemsolving behaviour as a function of personality drive and practice. Unpublished doctoral Thesis, Punjab University, Chandigarh, India.

Kumar, G, (1978) Creativity functioning in relation to personality, value orientation and achievement motivation. *Indian Educational Review*, 13(2), 110-115.

Kumar, D. and Kapila, A. (1987) Problem solving as a function of extraversion and masculinity, *Personality and Individual differences*, 8, 129-132.

Kumar, D, and Kumari, S. (1988) Problem solving as a function of creativity and personality. *Psychological Studies*, 33(3).

Kundu, D. (1986) A study of creativity, ego-strength, and extraversion: An empirical investigation, *Indian Dissertation Abstracts*, XV (1–2), 165–168.

Kundu, R. and Mallick, M.B. (1987) Environmental impact on creative production. Indian Journal of Community Guidance Service, 4(3), 55–61.

Kuppuswamy, B. (1976) *A Test Book of Child Behaviour and Development*. Delhi Vikas Publishing House Pvt. Ltd., P. 111.

Kurtzman, K.A. (1967) A study of school attitude, peer acceptance and personality of creative adolescents. *Exceptional Children*, 34(3), 157-162.

Lajoie, S.P. and Shore, B.M. (1987) Impulsivıty, reflectivity and high IQ. *Gifted Education International Abstract*, 493), 139-141.

Loasa, L.M. (1980) Maternal teaching strategies in Chicano and Anglo-American families. The influence of culture and education on maternal behaviour. *Child Development.*, 51, 759-765.

Loasa, L.M. and DeAvila, E.A. (1979) Development of cognitive styles among Chicanos in traditional and dualistic communities. *International Journal of Psychology*, 14, 91-98.

Laosa, L.M. and Sigel, I.E. (1982) *Families as Learning Environments for Children*, New York: Plenum.

Larsen, W.W. (1980) Cognitive tempo and intellectual peformance in college students. *Psychological Reports*, 47, 989-990.

Lefcourt, H.M. (1966) Inernal vs. external control of reinforcement: A review, *Psychological Bulletin*, 65, 206-220.

Linn, M.C. (1978) Influence of cognitive style and training on task requiring sepration of variables schema, *Child Development*, 49, 874-877.

Long, G.M. (1974) Reported correlates of perceptual style: a review of the field dependence/independency/dimension. *JSAS Catalog of Selected Documents in Psychology*, 4, 403, (Ms. No. 540).

Lorr, M, and Jenkins, R.L. (1953) Three factors in parent behaviour *Journal of Consulting Psychology*, 17, 306-308.

Maccoby, E.D. and Jacklin, C.N. (1974) *The Psychology of Sex Differences*, Stanford University Press, Stanford.

MacGregor, M. and Smith, J.L. (1965) Originality and role perception in elementary and junior high school children. *Dissertation Abstracts*, 25,6762.

Mackinnon, D.W. (1962) What makes a person creative? *Saturday Review*, 46(6), 15-17.

Mackinnon, D.W. (1964) The creativity of Architects. In Taylors (Ed.), *Widening Horizons in Creativity*, N.Y. Wiley.

Mackinnon, D.W. (1965) Personality and realization of creative potential. *American Psychologist*, 28, 273-281.

Majundar, D.N. (1950) *The Affairs of a Tribe: A Study in Tribal Dynamics*, Universal Publishers Ltd., Lucknow.

Melhara, S.B. (1985) Developing Creativity, the essential human trait. *Journal of Indian Education* , March, 9-14.

Mallapa, K.R. and Upadhyaya, R. (1977) Creativity and personality *Indian Psychological Review*, 14(2), 31-35.

Manjuvani, E. (1989) Influence of Home and School environment on Mental health Status of Children. Ph. D. thesis S. V. University

Marcias, J. (1987) The hidden curiculum of papago teachers : American Indian strategies for mitigating cultural discontinuity in early schooling. In G. Spindler and L. Spindler (Eds), *Interpretive Ethnography of Educatioin : At Home and Abroad*, Hillsdale, NJ: Erbaum, 363-380.

Mar I, S.K. (1971) Creativity of American and Arab rural youth: a cross cultural study, *Dissertation Abstracts International*, 31, 6407-A.

Majoribanks, K.(1978) Ethnicity, Family environment and cognitive performance. *Psychological Reports*, 42, 1277-1278.

Marx, R.W., Howard, D.C. and Winne, P.H. (1987) Student's perception of instruction, cognitive style and achievement. *Perceptual and Motor Skills*, 65, 123–134.

Massari, D.J. (1975) The relation of reflection-impulsivity to field dependence/independence and internal-external control in children, *Journal of Genetic Psychology*, 126, 61-67.

Mathur, R.N. and George, K.J. (1985) Nurturing creativity through individually guided system of instruction. *Journal of Indian Education*, November, 31-32.

Matthews, G. (1986) The effects of anxiety on intellectual peformance when and why are they found ? *Journal of Research in Personality*, 20(4), 386-410.

Mcshane, D (1983) Explaining achievement patterns of American Indian children. A transcultural and development model. *Peabody Journal of Education*, 61,34-48.

Mcshare, D, (1988) An analysis of mental health research with American Indian youth. *Journal of Adolescence*, 11, 87-116.

Mcshare, D. and Berry, J.W. (1986) Native North Americans: Indian and Inuit abilites. In J.H. Irvine and J.W. Berry (Eds). *Human abilities in Cultural Context*, Cambridge: Cambridge University Press, 385-426.

Mcshane, D. and Cook, V. (1985) Transcultural intellectual assessment: Hispanic performance on the wechslers. In B. Wolman (Ed) *Hand Book of Intelligence. Therories, Measurements and Application*, New York: Wiley.

McWhinnie, H.J. (1967) Some relationship between creativity and perception and in sixth grade children. *Perceptual and Motor Skills*, 25, 979-980.

Meddinus, G. and Love, J.M. (1965) The relation between curiosity and security in preschool children. *Journal of Genetic Psychology*, 107, 91-98.

Mednic, S.A. (1962) The associative basis of the creative process, *Psychological Review*, 69, 220-232.

Mehdi, B. (1973) *Manual of Verbal and Non-Verbal Tests of Creative Thinking*, Aligarh. India: Mrs. Qumar Fatima.

Mehdi, B. (1977) Creativity, intelligence and achievement, a correlational study. *Psychological Studies*, 22(1), 55-62.

Messer, S. (1970) The effect of anxiety over intellectual performance on reflection/impulsivity in children. *Child Development*, 41, 723-735.

Messer, S.B. (1972) The relation to internal-external control to academic performance. *Child Development*, 43, 1456-1462.

Messer, S.B. and Brodzinsky, D.M. (1979) The relation of conceptual tempo to aggression and its control. *Child Development*, 50(1), 758-766.

Messick, S. and Damarin, F. (1964) Cognitive style and memory for faces, *Journal of Abnormal and Social Psychology*, 69, 313-318.

Middents, G.J. (1968) The relationship of creativity and anxiety. *Dissertation Abstracts*, 28, 2526-A.

Miller, A.S (1953) An investigation of some hypothetical relationships of rigidity and strength and speed of perceptual closure. Unpublished doctrol dissertation. University of California.

Misra, K.S. (1986) *Effect of Home and School Environment on Scientific Creativity*. Snagyanalaya, Kanpur.

Mohaptra, K. (1980) cognitive abilites of unschooled tribal children and interethnic comparative analysis of the Bonda and The Dongria Kandh of Orissa, *Proceedings, of the 5th International conference of the International Association for Cross Cultural Studies*. Bhubaneswar.

Moore, S.C. and Bulbulian, K.N. (1976) The effects of contrasting styles of adult-child interaction on children's curiosity. *Developmental Psychology*, 12(2), 171-172.

Morgan, C.K. Richard, A.W., John, R. and Schopler, J. (1986) *Introduction to Psychology*, McGraw Hill Book company, Singapore, 136-161.

Morris, T.L. and Bergum B.O. (1978) A note of the relationship between field independence and creativity, *Perceptual and Motor Skills*, 46, 1114.

Muddu, V. (1980) A study of some personality correlates of intelligence and creative abilities among high school students in Andhra Pradesh, Ph.D. (Education), Thesis, Osmania Univesity.

Nair, P.M. (1975) Personality characteristics of creativie high school students. Ph. D. (Education) Thesis, Kerala University.

Nair, S. and Babu, N. (1977) A factor analytical comparison of personality variables related to high and low creative thinkers. Quest in Education, 14(1) 54-63.

Narmada, R. (1972) *Health of the pre school child*. Indian Association for Pre School Education, New Delhi, p.90.

Neufield, J.J. (1964) The relationship of creative thinking abilities to the academic achievement of adolescents. *Dissertation Abstracts*, 25, 3404.

Newland, G.A. (1981) Differences between left and right handedness on a measure of creativity, *Perceptual and Motor Skills*, 53, 787-792.

Nichols, R.C. (1964) Parental attitudes of mothers of intelligent adolescents and creativity of their children, *Child Development*, 35, 1041-1050.

Nijhawan, H.K. (1971) Anxiety in School Children, New Delhi : Wiley Eastern Private Ltd.

Noppe, L.D. (1977) A cognitive style approach to creative thought. *Journal of Personality Assessment*, 41, 85-90.

Nowicki, S. (1977) *A Manual for the Children's Nowicki-Stick Land: Internal-External Control Scale*, Unpublished Manuscript, Emory

University.

Nowicki, S, and Duke, M.P. (1974) A locus of control scale for college and non-college adults, *Journal of Personality Assessment*, 38, 136-137.

Nowicki, S. and Strickland, B.R. (1973) A locus of control scale for children, *Journal of Consulting and Clinical Phychology*, 40, 148-155.

Nuttla, E.V. (1969) Creativity in boys: A study of the influence of social background, educational achievement and parental attitudes on the creative behaviour of ten year old boys. *Dissertaion Abstracts International*, 31 (IA), 213.

Ogletree, E.J. (1968) A cross-cultural exploratory study of the creativeness of Steiner and State school pupils in England, Scotland and Germany. *Dissertation Abstracts*, 29, 516-A.

Ogletree, E.J. and Ujlaki, W. (1973) Effects of social class status on tests on creative behaviour. *Journal of Educational Research*, 67(4), 149-152.

Okonji, O.M. (1969) The differential effects of rural and urban upbringing on the development of cognitive styles. *International Journal of Psychology*, 4, 293–305.

O'Leary, M.R., Calsyn, D.A. and Fauria, T. (1980) The Group Exbedded Figures Test, *Journal of Personality Assessment*, 4, 532-537.

Olshin, G.M. (1965) The relationship among selected subject variables and levels of creativity. Unpublished doctoral thesis, University of Georgia, Athons.

Olton, (1969) The development of productive thinking skills in fifth grade children. *Research in Education*, 4, Ed, 021312.

Orcutt, L. (1968) Conformity tendencies among three and five year olds in an impersonal situational task. Psychological Reports, 23,387-390.

Orienstein, A.S. (1961) An investigation of Parental child-rearing attitudes and creativity in children. Doctrol Dissertation. University of Denver, Denver, Colorado, (Unpublished).

Osborne, B. (1985) Research into native north American's Cognition

1973-1982. *Journal of American Indian Education*, 24, 9-25.

Overall, J.E. and Klett, C.J. (1972) *Applied Multivariate Analysis*, MacGraw-Hill, New York.

Panek, E.P. (1982) Relationship between field dependence/independence and personality in order adult females. *Perceptual and Motor Skills*, 54, 811-814.

Panucci, M.R. (1978) The relationship of sex and ethnicity to anxiety, self-concept and creativity among continuation high school students. *Dissertation Abstracts International*, 38, 4056.

Paramesh, C.R. (1970) Value Orientations of Creative Persons. *Psychological Studies*, 15, 108-112.

Paramesh, C.R.(1971) Adaptation of Wallach and Kogan Creativity instruments and the relationship between creativity and intelligence. *Indian Journal of Psychology*, 46(1), 1-11.

Paramesh, C.R. (1972) *Creativity and Personality*. Madras, Janata Book Company, 163.

Paramesh, C.R. and Narayan, S. (1976) Effect of Creativity and intelligence on temperament. *Psychological Studies*, 21(2), 55-57.

Parloff, M. and Datta, L. (1966) personality characteristics of the potentially creative scientists. In J.H. Maserman (Ed). Schience and *Psychoanalysis*, 8, 91-96.

Passi, B.K. (1972) An exploratory study of creativity and its relationship with intelligence and achievement in school subjects at higher secondary stage, Ph, D. (Unpublished) Punjab University, Chandigarh, In *Indian Dissertation Abstracts*, 1975.

Passi, B.K. and Lalitha, M.S. (1975) A factorial study of creativity, intelligence, and self-concept of adolescents. *Psychological Stuides*, 20(1), 50-55.

Patel, K. (1976) Profiles of creative personality. *Psychologia : An International Journal of Psychology in the Orient*, 19(4), 173-183.

Paul, S. (1986) A study of cognitive styles of high school students of Home Science in relation to age, achievement, home environ-

ment and social class. University of Agra, *Indian Dissertation Abstracts*, Vol. XVI, No. 3, 1987, 347-358.

Payne, D.A., Helpin W.G., Ellett, C.D. and Dale, J.B. (1975) General Personality correlates of creative personality in academically and artistically gifted youth. *Journal of Special Education*, 9(1), 105-108.

Pedersen, D.M. (1965) Ego strength and discrepancy between conscious and unconscious self-concepts. *Perceptual and Motor Skills*, 20, 691-692.

Pedersen, F.A. and Wender, P.H. (1968) Early social correlates of cognitive functioning in six-year-old boys. *Child Development*, 39, 186-193.

Peters, M.F. (1988) Parenting in black families with young children : A historical perspective. In H.P> McAdoo (Ed) *Black Families*, Beverly Hills, Ca: Sage, 2nd ed, 228-241.

Phares, E.J. (1957) Expectancy changes in skill and chance situations, *Journal of Abnormal and Social Psychology*, 339-342.

Phatak, P. (1962) Experimental study of creativity and intelligence and school achievements. *Psychological Studies*, 7, 1-9.

Phillips, V.K. (1973) Creativity : Performance, profiles and perceptions. *The Journal of Psychology*, 83, 25-30.

Phillips, V.K. and Torrance, E.P. (1971) Divergent thinking, remote association and concept attainment strategies. *Journal of Psychology*, 77, 223-228.

Piaget, J, (1963) *The Psychology of Intelligence*, London, Routledge.

Piaget, J. (1967) *Six Psychological Studies*, New York : Random house.

Piaget, J. (1971) The theory of stages in cognitive development. In Green, D., Ford, K. and Flamer, G., (Eds.) *Measurement and Piaget*, New Yrok : McGraw Hill, 1-11.

Piers, E.V., Danies, J.M. and Quacken, B.J.F. (1960) The identification of creativity in adolescents. *Journal of Educational Psychology*, 51, 346-351.

Powell, G.J., Morales, A., Romero, A. and Yamamoto, J. (Eds) (1983) *The Psycholosocial Development of Minority Group Children*,

New York : Bruner/Mazel.

Prakash, A.O. (1966) Understanding the fourth grade slump : A study of the creative thinking abilities of Indian children.Master's Thesis, University of Minnesota (Unpublished).

Partap, D.R. (1968) *The Banjaras of Bapunagar (A Settlement in the Urban Environs of Hyderabad)*, A.P. Tribal Culture Research and Training Institute.

Punetha, D.(1980) Socialization of Aggression in children in a tribal society. In Sinha, D. (Ed) *Socialization of the Indian Child*, 102-117.

Rai, S.(1982) Problem solving in science of creative and non-creative students, Ph. D. (Education) Thesis, Patna University.

Raina, M.K. (1969) A study of some correlates of creativity in Indian students. Unpublished Doctoral dissertation, University of Rajasthan.

Raina, M.K. (1969) A study of sex difference in creativity in India. *Journal of Creative Behaviour*, 3, 111-114.

Raina, M.K (1970) A study of creativity in teachers, *Psychological Studies*, 15.

Raina, M.K. (1971) Verbal and non-verbal creative thinking ability: A study of sex differences. *Journal of Education and Psychology*, 29, 175-180.

Raina, T.N. (1980) Sex differences in creativity in India. A second book. *The Journal of Creative Behaviour*, 14, 218-219.

Raman, E.J. (1971) Discriminant Function Analysis - A technique for classification. *Journal of Psychological Research*, 15, 37-38.

Ramirez, M. (1983) *Psychology of the Americans*. Elmsford, NY : Pergamon.

Ramirez, M. and Castaneda, A. (1974) *Cultural Democracy Bicognitive Development, and Education*, New York : Academic Press

Rastogi, M. (1987) A Study of Cognitive of style in relation to intelligence and creativity. *Journal of Personality and Clinical Studies*, 3(2), 161-164.

Rastogi, M. and Nathawat, S.S. (1982) effect of creativity on mental health, *Psychological Studies*, 27(2) 74-76.

Rawat, M.S. and Agarwal, s. (1977) A study on creative thinking with reference to intelligence, age, sex, communities and income groups. *Indian Psycholgical Review*, 1292), 36-40.

Razik, T.M.A. (1964) An investigation of creative thinking among college students. *Dissertation Abstracts*, 24, 2775.

Richmond, B.O. (1971) Creative and cognitive and abilities of white and Negro children. *Journal of Negro Education*, 40(2).

Richmond, B.O. and Serna, M.D.L. (1980) Creativity and locus of control among Mexican college students. *Psychological Reports*, 46, 979-983.

Roe A. (1960) Crucial life experience in the development of scientists. In Torrance E.P. (Ed.) *Talent and Educatioin. Minneapolis*, Minnesota University of Minnesota Press, 66-77.

Rogers, D. (1962) *Child Psychology*, California, Belmont : Brooks Cole Publishing Company, p. 159.

Rosen, B. and D' Andrade, R. (1959) The psychological origins of achievements motivation. *Sociometry*, 22, 185-218.

Rotter, J.B. (1966) Generalized expectancies for internal vs. external control of re-inforcement, *Psychological Monographs*, 80, 609.

Rotter, J.B. and Mulry,R.(1965) Internal versus external control of reinforcements and decision time. *Journal of Personality and Social Psychology*, 2, 599-604.

Sachidananda and Mukhopadhyay, K.L.(1965) *Profiles of Tribal Cultural in Bihar,* Calcuatta, p. 38.

Sagar, C.J. and Kaplan H.S. (1972) *Progress in Group and Family Therapy*, New York : Brunner Mazel

Salkind, N.J , Kojima, H. and Zelniker, T.(1978) Cognitive tempo in American, Japanese and Israeli children. *Child Development*, 49, 1024-1027.

Salkind, N.T. and Wright, J.C. (1977) The development of reflection-impulsivity and cognitive efficiency, *Human development*. 20,377-387.

Saracho, O.N. (1983) Cultural differnces in the cognitive style of Mexican-American students. *Journal of the Association for the study of Perception, International*, 18(1), 3-10.

Saran, V. (1970) A study of personality traits of nursery school children against the background of their home environment, Doctrol thesis, University of Agra.

Seveca, A.F. (1965) The effects of reward, race, IQ and socio-economic status on creative production of pre school children. Unpublished doctrol dissertion, Louisiana State University, Baton Rouge, Louisicana.

Saxena, M. and Sharma, V.K. (1986) An empirical investigation of adjustment patterns of high low creative adolescents. *Manas*, 33 (1–2), 65-73.

Schlefier, M. and Douglas, V. (1973) Moral judgements behaviour and cognitive style in young children. *Canadian Journal of Negro Education*, 56, 21-34.

Scott-Jones, D. (1987) Mother-as-teacher in the families of high and low achieving, low income black first graders. *Journal of Negro Education*, 56, 21-34.

Seifert, K.L. and Hoffnung, R.J. (1987) *Child and Adolescent Development*, Boston, : Houghton Mifflin.

Shade, B.J. (1986) Is there an Afro-American cognitive styles? An exploratory study. *Journal of Black Psychology*, 13(1) 13-16.

Shainess, N, (1989) The roots of creativity. *American Journal of Psychoanalysis*, 49(2), 127-138.

Sharma, K.N. (1972) Rural-urban differences in creative thinking. *Journal of Psychological Research*, 16, 121-122.

Sharma, K.N. (1974) Creativity as a function of intelligence interests and culture. *Creativity News Letter*, 3, 30-37.

Sharma, K.N. (1981) A study of intrinsic value structures and creativity among higher secondary school girls. *Journal of Psychological Research*, 25(1), 1-4.

Sharma, A. and Sharma, (1987) Creativity, intelligent and socio-economic status, *Indian Educational Review*, 17(1), 64-68.

Shipe, D. (1971) Impulsivity and lucus of contol as predictors of achievement and adjustment in mildly retarted and borderline youth. *American Journal of Mental Deficiency*, 76, 12-22.

Shmukler, DE. (1982-83) Early home background features in relation to imaginative and creative expression in third grade. Imagination, Cognition and personality, 2(4), 311-321. In *Psychological Abstracts*, 1984, 71(6), 1543.

Shon, S.P. and Ja, D.Y., (1983) Asian families, In M. McGoldric, J.K. Pearce and J. Giordano (Eds), *Ethnicity and Family Therapy*, New York: Guliford.

Shukla, J.P. and Sharma, V.P. (1986) Sex differences in Scientific creativity, Indian *Psychological Review*, 30(3), 32-35.

Siddamma, T. (1979) A study of certain behavioral determinants of obesity children. Ph. D. thesis, S.V. University.

Siegel, A.W. Kirasic, K.C. and Klourg, R.R. (1973) Recognition memeory in reflective and impulsive pre school children. *Child Development*, 44, 651-656.

Sigg, J, and Gargiulo, R. (1980) Creativity and cognitive style in learning disabled and nondisabled school age children, *Psychological Reports*, 46, 299-305.

Silverberg, R.A. (1970) The relationship of children's perceptions of parental behaviour to the creativity of their children *Dissertation Abstracts International*, 31(12-A).

Simpkins, R, and Eisenman, R. (1968) Sex differences in creativity. *Psychological Reports*, 22, 996.

Singer, J.L. (1961) Imagination and writing ability in young children. *Journal of Personality*, 29, 396-413.

Singer D.L. and Rummo, J. (1973) Ideational creativity and behaviour style in kindergarden age children. *Developmental Psychology*, 8, 154-161.

Singh, C.P. (1971) Creative Abilities : Cross-Cultural Study. IBSA, 2(2), 208.

Singh, O.P. (1982) A study of creativity of high school students in relation to intelligence and socio-economic status, Ph, D. (Education) Thesis, Avadh University.

Singh, R.P. (1977) Education for creativity, Indian *Psychological Review*, 1492), 67-68.

Singh R.P. (1978) Divergent thinking abilities and creative personality dimensioins of bright adolescent boys and girls. *Indian Educational Review*, 13(4), 82-91.

Singh, R.P. (1981) Creativity in relation to adjustment. *Psychological Studies* 26(2), 84-85.

Singh, R.P. (1981) A study of creativity as function of adjustment, frustration and level of aspiration. *Indian psychological Review*, 20(4), 39-42.

Singh, S.K. (1970) Group Structure and creatie functioining, *Indian psychological Review*, 14, 11-15.

Sinha, N.C.P. and Sharma, M (1978) Creativity and adjustment. *Indian Psychological Review*, 1692), 4-7.

Slughter, D.T. and Epps, E.G. (1987) Home environment and academic achievement of black Amercian children and youth: An overview. *Journal of Negro Education*, 56,3-20.

Smilansky, J, and Halberstadt, N.(1986) Inventory vs. problem solvers, *The Journal of Creative Behaviour*, 20, 183-210.

Smith, R. (1965) *Relation of Creativity to Social Class, Co-operative Research Project*, No. 2250, University of Pittsbergh, 90-93.

Smith, R.M. (1965) *Creativity and Socio-economic status in Indian Research on Creativity*. Agra Psychological research Cell, Agra.

Smith, T. V. (1971) Acculturation and field dependence among the Xhosa, *Journal of Behavioural Science*, 1(3), 121-123.

Smith J. D. and Caplan, J. (1988) Cultural differences in cognitive style development. *Developmental Psychology*, 249(1), 46-52.

Smith, T.P. and Ribordy, S.C. (1980) Correlates of reflection-impulsivity in Kindergarden males: Intelligence, scio-economic status, race, father's absence, and teacher's ratings. *Psychological Reports*, 47, 1187-1191.

Solomon, A.O, (1968) A comparative analysis of creative and intelligent behaviour of elementary school children with different socio-economic background. *Dissertation Abstracts*, 29, 1457 A.

Sorenson, H., Malm, N, and Forehand, G.A. (1975) *Psychology of Learning*, Tata McGraw Hill Publishing Company, New Delhi.

Sowjanya, K (1974) Creativity of preadolescents influence of shcool, home, socio-economic status, sex and age, M.Sc. dissertation, S.V. University.

Spindler, G. and Spindler, L. (1987) *Interpretive Ethnography of Education*, Hillsdale, NJ : Erlbaum.

Spotts, J.V. and Mackler, B., (1967) Relationships of field dependent and field-independent cognitive style of creative test performance. *Perceptual and Motor Skills*, 24,239-268. (Monogr. Suppl. 2-V24).

Srichandra, (1970) Scientist; *A Social and Psychological Study*, Bombay, Oxford and Indian Book House.

Srinivas, H.N. (1962) *Caste in Modern India and Other Essays*, New York : Asia Publishihng House, P.3.

Stein, M.I. (1953) Creativity and Culture, *Journal of Psychology*, 36, 311-322.

Stein, M.I. (1963) A transactional approach to creativity. In Taylor, C.W. and Barron, F. (Eds.) *Scientific Creativity: Its Recognition and Development*. New York : John Wiley, 217-227.

Steward, M. and Steward, D (1973) The observation of Anglo-Mexican and Chinese-American mothers teaching their young sons. *Child Development*, 44, 339-337.

Straus, M.E. and Straus, M.A. (1968) Family roles and sex differences in creativity of children in Bombay and Minneapolis, *Journal of Marriage and Family*, 30,46-53.

Sumangala, V. (1987) Intelligence and social adjustment as predictors of creativity among secondary school pupils. *Experiments in Education*, 211-216.

Sundararaj, N. (1959) The Discriminant Function Analysis: Its technique and use in psychology and psychiatry. *Journal of the All India Institute of Mental Health*, Bangalore, 2(1).

Swan, R.W. and Stavros, H. (1973) child rearing practices associated with the development of the cognitive skills of children in low socio-economic areas. *Early Child Development and Care*, 2(1), 23-28.

Symonds, P.M. (1939) *The Psychology of Parent-child Relationship*, New York : Appleton Century Crafts.

Tara, S.N. (1981) Sex differences in creativity among early adolescents in India. *Perceptual and Motor Skills*, 5, 959-962.

Taylor, C.H. (1964) *Widening Horizons in Creativity*. New York: Wilely.

Terman, L.M. (1954) The discovery and encouragement of exceptional talent. *American Psychologist*, 9, 221-230.

Terman, L.M. (1959) The gifted group at mid-life, thirty five years follow-up of the superior child. *Genetic studies of Genius. Stanford*, California, Stanford University Press 5.

Tharakan, P.N.O, (1987) The effect of rural and urban upbringing on cognitive styles. *Psychological Studies*, 32(2).

Thoman, W.A.M. (1971) The role of cognitive style variables in mediating the influence of aggressive televison upon elementary school children. unpublished dectoral dissertation, University of California, Los Analges.

Thurston, E. (1906) *Castes and Tribes of Southern India* (Vols. I-VII). Madras Government Press, Madras.

Torrance E.P. (1962) *Guiding Creative Talent*. N.J. Prentice Hall, Englewood, Cliffs.

Torrance, E.P. (1962) *Education and creative Potential*, Minneapolis University of Minnesota Press.

Torrance, E.P. (1964) Education and Creativity. In C.W. Taylor (Ed.) *Creativity: Progress and Potential*. Mc-Graw-Hill, New York, 50-128.

Torrance, E.P. (1967) *Torrance Test of Creative Thinking: Norms Technical Manual*, New Jersey: Personnel Press Inc.

Torrance, E.P. (1967) *Understanding the Frouth Grade Slump in Creative Thinking*. Final report on cooperative research Project, N. 994, United States Office of Education, University of Georgia, Athens.

Torrance, E.P. (1968) A longitudinal Examination of the fourth grade slump in creativity. *Gifted Child Quarterly*, 12(4), 195-199.

Torrance, E.P. (1969) What is honored: Comparative studies of creative achievement and motivation. *The Journal of Creative Behaviour*, 3, 149-154.

Torrance, E.P. and Aliotti, N.C. (1969) Sex differnces in levels of performance and test-retest reliability on the Torrance Test of Creative Thinking abilaity. *Journal of Creative Behaviour*.

Tripathi, D.K.M. and Tripathi, N.K.M. (1984) perceptual dependence in relation to approval motive, socio-economic status and locus of control. *Psychological Studies*, 29(10) 60-63.

Trowbridge, N. (1968) Cross-cultural study of creative ideas in children, *Comparative Education Review*, 12, 80-83.

Trowbridge, N and Charles, D.C. (1966) Creativity in art students. *Journal of Genetic Psychology*, 109, 281-289.

Tuli, M. (1982) Sex and regional differences in mathematical creativity. *Indian Educational Review*, 17, 128-134.

Ulahambal, S.(1984) personality traits of adolescents, *Abstracts of Research Studies*, 1980-85, Sri Avinashilingam Home Science, College, Coimbatore, p.8.

Vaught, G,.M. (1965) The relationship of role identification and ego strength to sex differences in the Rod-and-Frame Test, *Journal of Personality*, 33(2), 271–282.

Vectoria, N.B. (1980) Verbal instruction and personality factors in perceptual peformance, *Revista de Psychologie*, 269(2), 161-168.

Venkata Rami Reddy, A, and Balakrishan Reddy, P. (1983) Creativity and intelligence, *Psychological Studies*. 28(1), 20-23.

Venkata Rami Reddy, A. and Balakrsihan Reddy, P (1981) Creativity of adolescent boys and girls in relation to some variables. *Indian Education Review*, 17, 1-14.

Venkata Rami Reddy, A., and Saleema, K. (1988) Creativity vs. Age. *Pespectives in Education*, 4, 245-250.

Venkata Rami Reddy, A. and Tulasi Devi, S. (Unpublished) A study on sex differences in creativity. M.Ed. dissertation, S.V. University Tirupati.

Venkateswara Rao, R. (1987) Human resources-creativity. *Progressive Educational Herald*, 2, 46-50,53.

Vemon, P.E. (1972) *Intelligence and Culture Environment*. Methuen and Co., Ltd., 11, New Felter Lane London EC4 P4EF2.

Vernon, P.E. (1972) The distinctiveness of field independence. *Journal of Personality*, 40(30), 366-386.

Vygotsky, L.S (1978) *Mind in Society*, Cambridge, M.A. : Harward University Press.

Wade, SE. (1971) Adolescents, Creativity and Media. *American Behavioral Scientist*, 14, 341-351.

Walberg, H. D. (1971) Varieties of adolescent creativity and the high school environment. *Exceptional Children*, 38, 111-116.

Walker, P.C. (1969) A study of creativity among Mexican school children. Doctoral disertation, University of Georgia.

Wallach, M.A. and Kogan, N (1965) *Modes of thinking in Young Children*, New York; Holt.

Wallach, M.A. and Kogan, N. (1965) A new look at creativity intellgence distinction. *Journal of Personality*, 33, 348-369.

Ward, C.W. (1968) Reflection-impulsivity in Kindergarden children. *Child Development*, 39(3), 865-873.

Ward, J.(1968) Comment on an alternative towards factors analysis of Wallach and Kogan's "Creativity" correlation. *British Journal of Psychology*, 38, 331.

Ward, W.C. (1973) *Disadvantages Children and their First school Experiences: Development of Self-regulatory Behaviours* (PR-73-18), Princeton, J.J. : Educational Testi Service.

Ward, W.C. and Cox, P.W. (1974) A field study of non-verbal creativity. *Journal of Personality*, 42, 202-219.

Watsa, S. (1979) Creative Education. *Indian Psychological Review*, 18(1-4), Special Issues, 49-51.

Watson, G. (1957) Some personality difference in children related to strict or permissive parental discipline. *Journal of psychology*,

44, 227-249.

Weiner, A.S. and Berzonsky, M.D. (1975) Development of selective attention in reflective and impulsive children. *Child Development*, 46, 545-548.

Weintraub, S.A. (1973) Self-control as a correlate on an internalizing-externalizing symptom dimension. *Journal of Abnormal Child Psychology*, 1, 293-3-7.

Weisberg, P.S. and Springer, K.J. (1961) Environment factors in creative function: A study of gifted children. *Archives of General Psychiatry*, 5, 554-564.

Werner (1947) *Comparative Psychology of Mental Development*, New York, Follett.

White, K.P. (1947) Anxiety entroversion introversion and divergent thinking ability. *Journal of Creative Behaviour*, 2(2), 119-127.

Whiting, J.W.M. and Child, J.L. (1953) *Child Training and Personality*, New Haven: Yale Univesity Press.

Wiedl, K.H. and Bethge, H.J. (1981) The direct of regulation promoting situation changes on intelligence performance and looking behaviour of cognitive impulsive children. *Psychologie*, 13(2), 127-141.

Winterbottom, M, (1958) The relation of need for achievement in learning experience in independence and mastery. In Atkinson, J.(Ed.). *Motives in Fantacy Action and Society*, Princeton, J.J., Van Nostrand, 453-478.

Witkin, H.K. and Berry, J.W. (1975) Psychological differentiation in cross-cultural perspective. *Journal of Cross-cultural Psychology*, 6, 84-87.

Witkin, H.A. Dyk. R.B. Faterson, H.F., Goodenough, D.R. and Karp, S.A. (1962) *Psychological Differentiation*, New York, Wiley.

Witkin, H.A. Goodenough, D.R. and Karp, S.A. (1967) Stability of cognitive style from childhood to young adulthood. *Journal of Personality and Social Psychology*, 7(3), 291-300.

Witkin, H.A., Lewis, H.B., Hetzman, M., Machover, K., Meissner, P.B. and Wapner, S.(1954) *Personality through Perception*, New

York, Harper.

Witkin, H.A., Moore, C.A. Goodenough, D.R. and Cox, PIW. (1977) Field-dependent and field-independent cognitive styles and their educational implications, *Review of Educational Research*, 47, 61-64.

Witt, O.C. (1955). Sex differences in Perception, Unpublished Master's Thesis, University of Utrecht.

Wober, M. (1967) Adapting Witkin's field independence theory to accomodate new information from Africa. *British Journal of Psychology*, 58, 29-38.

Woerner and Levine (1950) (Unpublished) Cited by Goodenough, D.R. and Karp, S.A. (1961) Field dependence and intellectual functioning. *Journal of Abnormal and Social Psychology*, 63(2), 241-246.

Wolf, R. (1941) The measurement of environment. In Anastasi, A. (Ed.). *Testing Problems is Perspective*. Washington, D.C., American council on Education, 1966.

Wolters, B.J. (1976) The Creative Personality (Duth) *Gedrag: Tijchrift voor Psychologie* 3(6), 348-361 (abstract).

Wrigght, C. (1987) Nuturing crative potential: An interactive model for home and school. *Creative Child and Adult Quarterly*, 12(1), 31-38.

Wright, J.C. (1973) *The KRISP : A Technical Report*. Unpublished manuscript, (Available from J.C. Wright, Kanas Center for Research in Early Childgood Education, University of Kanas, Lawarence, Kanas).

Yadav, A.N. and Dash, A.S. (1980) Cognitive-affective abilities and social background of tribal and non-tribal primary school drop-outs. Utkal University, M.Phil. Thesis (Unpublished).

Young, H.H,. Jr. (1959) A test of Witkin's field dependence hypothesis, *Journal of Abnormal Social Psychology*, 59, 188-192.

Young, M. and McGreeney, P. (1968) *Learning Begins at Home*. London: Routlege and Kegan Paul, 16.

Zuckman, L. (1957) Hysteric-compulsive factors in personality organization. Unpublished Doctoral Dissetation. New School of Social Research.

Index

Young, 24, 66, 150